Daniel D. Slade

Diphtheria, its nature and treatment

With an account of the history of its prevalence in various countries

Daniel D. Slade

Diphtheria, its nature and treatment
With an account of the history of its prevalence in various countries

ISBN/EAN: 9783742826961

Manufactured in Europe, USA, Canada, Australia, Japa

Cover: Foto ©Lupo / pixelio.de

Manufactured and distributed by brebook publishing software
(www.brebook.com)

Daniel D. Slade

Diphtheria, its nature and treatment

WITH

AN ACCOUNT OF THE HISTORY OF ITS PREVALENCE
IN VARIOUS COUNTRIES.

BY

DANIEL D. SLADE, M. D.

BEING A SECOND AND REVISED EDITION OF AN ESSAY TO WHICH
WAS AWARDED THE FISKE FUND PRIZE OF 1860.

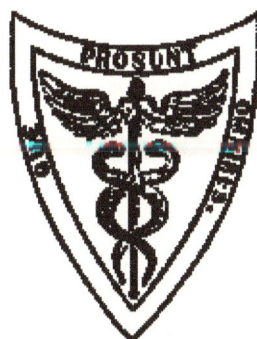

PHILADELPHIA:
BLANCHARD AND L
1864.

PHILADELPHIA:
COLLINS, PRINTER.

PREFACE.

THE publication of another edition of this essay has afforded an opportunity for its thorough revisal, and for such additions as experience and observation have taught us. Our knowledge of the nature, causes, and treatment of diphtheria is still lamentably deficient, and it is only by the most diligent study, and by the most careful observation, that we may hope to arrive hereafter at more satisfactory results.

BOSTON, *October*, 1864.

DIPHTHERIA.

No diseases of late years have awakened more attention, both among the profession and the public generally, than those which have been classed, more or less
correctly, under the term diphtheritic. Nor is this to be
wondered at when we consider the distressing nature of
the symptoms, and the terrible fatality with which the
epidemics of malignant sore throat have so often been
attended.

Diphtheria is a synonyme of the word Diphtherite,[1]
originally used by M. Bretonneau in his treatise on this
subject, which appeared in 1826, and which is chiefly
made up of his own observations on the epidemics of
malignant sore throat prevailing at Tours and in its
neighborhood in 1818, and again in 1825 and 1826.

The following are the specific characters of diphtherite,
according to M. Bretonneau :—[2]

At the commencement of the disease a circumscribed

---

[1] Διφθίρα and Διφθίρίς have both the same signification, the pre-
pared skin of an animal; Διφθίρίτις and Διφθίρίας both signify that
which is covered with skin.

[2] Traité de la Diphthérite, Paris, 1826, p. 49.

2

redness is seen, covered with a semitransparent coagu-
lated mucus. This first layer, which is slight, supple,
and porous, may be still further raised up by portions
of unaltered mucus, in such a manner as to form vesicles.
Frequently the red spots perceptibly extend from one to
another, either by continuity or by contact, like a liquid
which is spread out upon a flat surface, or which runs
by streaks in a tube. The concretion becomes opaque,
white, and thick, and assumes a membranous consistence.
In this stage it is easily detached, and does not adhere
to the mucous membrane, except by some very delicate
prolongations of concrete matter which penetrate into
the muciparous follicles. The surface which it covers is
usually of a faint red tint, with points of a deeper red;
this tint is brighter at the periphery of the spots.

If the false membrane, in detaching itself, leaves the
mucous surface uncovered, the redness which the exudation has concealed returns, and the points of a deeper
red allow blood to transude. The exudation is renewed
and becomes more and more adherent at the points
which were first attacked; it often acquires a thickness
of several lines, and passes from a yellowish-white to a
brown-gray or black color. At the same time the
transudation of blood becomes still more free, and is the
source of those *stillicidia* which have been so generally
noted by authors. At this time the alteration of the
organic surfaces is more apparent than at the beginning;
often portions of concrete matter are effused into the
very substance of the mucous tissue. A slight erosion

and sometimes even ecchymoses are observed at those points which, by their situation, are exposed to friction, or from which the avulsion of the false eschars has been attempted. It is especially just at this period that the pellicles which are undergoing decomposition give out a foul odor. If they are circumscribed, the œdematous swelling of the surrounding cellular tissue makes them appear depressed, and from this appearance alone we might be led to believe that we had before us a foul ulcer with a considerable loss of substance. If, on the contrary, they are extended over large surfaces, they are partly detached, hang in shreds more or less decomposed, and simulate the appearance of the last stages of sphacelus. But when we open the bodies of those who, after some days of sickness, die of tracheal diphtherite, we shall find in the air-passages all the gradations of this inflammation from its first stage on the portions recently attacked, up to that which by the aspect of a gangrenous alteration at the points which were first affected, is most likely to deceive us.

Diphtheria, according to M. Bretonneau, is a specific disease. Its specific character consists, anatomically, in the formation of a false membrane of definite structure —pathologically, in the power of reproducing itself. "Nothing is diphtheria that has not a pellicular exudation; no such exudation is diphtherical which is not capable of acting as a virus or contagion."

These were the views expressed in the treatise of M.

Bretonneau, and to these he still adheres, with some modifications, in a paper published in the *Archives Générales de Médecine*, 1855.

Under the term diphtheria, Bretonneau, however, has connected several affections, which in the prevailing nosology are separated from each other by wide intervals. This point will demand of us especial consideration.

How far his description of diphtheria is to be considered a faithful representation, how far it is to be taken as a universal type of the disease, are questions to be answered only by a careful comparison of the accounts of the epidemics of "sore throat" or "angina" which have invaded various portions of the world, at longer or shorter intervals, particularly during the last two centuries. On making such comparison it will be found that they exhibit marked differences in their characteristic symptoms and dangers, having been frequently regarded as different diseases. We shall, however, not only be satisfied of their identity, a fact so well established by Bretonneau, but also of the common character by which this identity may be recognized, viz., the existence of the exudation of false membrane.

As regards the special virulence of the diphtheritic exudation which constitutes an important feature in M. Bretonneau's views of diphtheria, it will be seen, as we proceed, that so far from inoculation being the only mode of propagation, there is no sufficient reason to suppose that a concrete virus exists; that epidemics of a rapidly fatal character have occurred, where the exudation has been extremely limited and where death has been brought about solely by the constitutional disturbance.

History.—We can undoubtedly trace back the history of this affection to a period almost contemporary with Homer. Whether such be the case or not, certain it is that, ten centuries later, we find distinct descriptions of a form of malignant sore throat in the writings of Aretæus, under the name of Egyptian or Syrian ulcer. This prevailed in the two countries, more especially among children. It was characterized by the appearance of ulceration in the throat, by fetid breath, and sometimes by great dyspnœa.

Macrobius speaks of a similar epidemic at Rome, A.D. 380, during which sacrifices were offered up to a certain Goddess—"ut populus Romanus, morbo, qui angina dicitur, promisso voto, sit liberatus."

A fatal epidemic of sore throat occurred in Holland, in 1337. Hecker,[1] in his account of the "Sweating sickness" of England, in 1517, says that—

"In January of that year, there appeared in Holland another disease which, from its dangerous and inexplicable symptoms, spread fear and horror around. It was a malignant and infectious inflammation of the throat, so rapid in its course that, unless assistance was procured within eight hours, the patient was past all

---

[1] Hecker's Epidemics, p. 224.

hope of recovery before the close of the day. Sudden pains in the throat, and violent oppression of the chest, especially in the region of the heart, threatened suffocation, and at length actually produced it. During the paroxysms the muscles of the throat and chest were seized with violent spasms, and there were but short intervals of alleviation, before a repetition of such seizures terminated in death. Unattended by any premonitory symptoms, the disease began with a severe catarrhal affection of the chest, which speedily advanced to inflammation of the air-passages.

"The physicians had recourse to venesection and purgatives. Moreover, the employment of detergent gargles, whereby the extension of the affection to the lungs was prevented, as also of demulcent pectoral remedies, was decidedly beneficial. . . Most of those affected were taken ill at the same time; and eleven days of suffering and misery had scarcely elapsed, when not another case occurred. It spread, however, no doubt, beyond Holland, for in the same year we find it in Basle, where, within eight months, it destroyed about 2000 people, and its symptoms would seem to have been more strongly marked.

"Respecting the intermediate countries, which it is highly probable that the disease passed through from Holland before it reached Basle, we unfortunately have no information. The tongue and gullet were white, as if covered with mould; the patient had an aversion to food and drink, and suffered from malignant fever,

accompanied with continued headache and delirium.
Here, in addition to an internal method of cure not detailed, the cleansing of the mouth was perceived to be
an essential part of the treatment; the viscous white
coating was removed every two hours, and the tongue
and fauces were afterwards smeared with honey of
roses."

In 1557, a similar epidemic appeared in Holland,
which proved very fatal, and which spread to other parts
of Europe. It has been described by M. Forest. He
says:—

"It was not so rapid in its course as in 1517, but
began with a slight fever, like a common catarrh, and
showed its great malignity only by degrees. Sudden
fits of suffocation then came on, and the pain of the
chest was so distressing that the patients imagined that
they must die in the paroxysm. The complaint was
increased still more by a tight convulsive cough. Death
did not take place till the ninth or fourteenth day. The
painful affection of the stomach was, in this epidemic,
very distinctly marked, so that a sense of pressure at the
precordia, accompanied by continued acid eructations,
continued to exist even after a succession of six or seven
fits of fever; and convalescents were troubled with dys-
pepsia, debility, and hypochondriasis."

In 1576, there was a very malignant form of throat
disease prevalent in Paris. In fact, from the end of the
16th century, we find that epidemics of angina have
shown themselves almost constantly to a greater or less

extent, in some portions of the old or new world. In the beginning of the 17th century, an epidemic of angina occurred in Spain, which received the name of "Garotillo," because those who were attacked by it perished as if strangled by a cord. This has been described by Mercatus, Villareal, Nunez, and by others. In 1618, the same disease appeared at Naples, which the inhabitants termed "male de canna," disease of the trachea. It raged here to a greater or less extent for twenty years, and has been described by several writers, among whom we may mention Nola, Carnevale, Syambati, Zacutus Lusitanus, and Marcus Aurelius Severinus. Carnevale, in particular, has given us full data of this epidemic in his treatise entitled, "De Epidemico Strangulatione Affectu." The children were first attacked, the disease afterwards spreading among the population generally, and proving very fatal. The disease commenced by a mild inflammation of the throat; soon the affected parts presented a whitish exudation; the breath became fetid; deglutition impossible; the respiration embarrassed, and the patient died of suffocation. This writer also gives us the different appearances which the pharynx presented in this epidemic; he also speaks of the extension of the disease to the trachea, œsophagus, pituitary membrane—of the diagnosis, prognosis, and the topical remedies, all of which are quite in accordance with modern views.

In 1632, Alaymus published a treatise upon "Syrian Ulcers." He prefers this term, he says, inasmuch as it applies to all forms of the disease, which he describes in a similar manner with Carnevale. No writer of this age, however, speaks of cutaneous diphtheria in connection with the other symptoms which they describe, although most of them particularly notice the extension of the disease to the air-passages.

From the middle of the seventeenth century up to 1740, we find but little mention made of the prevalence of malignant angina. But very shortly after this, in 1748, the disease made its appearance in Paris, where it prevailed until 1748, and has been described by Malouin and Chomel. At about the same time a similar epidemic appeared both in England and at Cremona, accounts of which are recorded by Fothergill, Starr, and Ghisi.

In England these epidemics proved very destructive. The epidemic described by Fothergill[1] is, without doubt, closely allied with scarlatina. He says:—

"It generally comes on with giddiness and chills, which are soon followed by great heat; these states alternate for a few hours, until, at length, the heat becomes constant and intense. Then follows acute pain in the head, heat and soreness, rather than pain of throat, stiffness of the neck, commonly great sickness or purging, or the two combined. The face soon after looks red and swelled, the eyes inflamed and watery, as in measles, restlessness, anxiety and faintness. If the mouth and throat be examined soon after the first attack,

---

[1] Account of the Sore Throat, attended with Ulcers. London, 1748.

the uvula and tonsils are found swelled; and these parts together with the velum palati and pharynx appear of a florid red color, which is most marked on posterior edge of palate in the angles above the tonsils, and upon the tonsils themselves. Instead of redness, a broad spot or patch of an irregular form and of pale white, is sometimes seen surrounded with florid red, which whiteness appears like that of the gums immediately after being pressed with the fingers, or as if matter ready to be discharged was contained beneath. Generally on the second day of the disease, the face, neck, breast and hands, are of a deep erysipelatous color, with a sensible tumefaction. A great number of small pimples of a color more intense than that which surrounds them appear on the arms and other parts. (In a note, he says, the eruption and redness have not so regularly accompanied the disease during the latter part of this winter, 1754, as they did last year. In some cases they did not appear at all, in others not till the third or fourth day.)

"The appearances in the fauces continue the same, except that the white places become more ash-colored; and it is now found that what might be taken for the superficial covering of a suppurated tumor is really a slough concealing an ulcer. Instead of the slough in mild cases, a superficial ulcer of an irregular form appears in one or more parts, scarce to be distinguished from the sound, but by the irregularity of surface which it occasions. Towards night heat and restlessness increase, and a peculiar kind of delirium frequently comes on. The pulse is generally very quick; in some, hard and small; in some, soft and full. The tongue is generally moist, and not often found. In some it is covered with a thick white fur; and these generally complain of soreness about the root of the tongue."

Fothergill also speaks of an acrid discharge from the nose, and remarks that there was sometimes epistaxis at the commencement of the attack. He describes faintness as a common symptom, also diarrhœa at the outset. He is very positive about the separation of sloughs which leave ulcers. Although he does not mention dropsy as a sequela, yet he evidently had entertained the notion of the disease being allied to scarlatina; but, he remarks, it differed from the sore throat and scarlet fever described in Edinburgh in 1733.

Ghisi, after having given a detailed description of the epidemic of sore throat which commenced at Cremona in 1747, remarks that the disease proved fatal by suffocation, even in those cases where the attention of the patient had not been called to the condition of the throat. This absence of difficulty in deglutition has been constantly observed, however, according to M. Bretonneau, in all the epidemics of malignant angina, particularly in those of Tours. Ghisi describes cases which appear to be primary and not secondary to scarlatina. He especially indicates the peculiarity of the pseudo-membranous concretion which lines the air-passages.

In 1747, M. Arnault, of Orleans, mentions cases of malignant sore throat which carried off the patient in twenty-four hours. At the autopsies of two children dead from this disease the mucous membrane of the trachea was found detached to the extent of several inches. It was of the consistence of parchment, and of a white color.

In 1768, Marteau de Grandvilliers published descriptions of cases of gangrenous angina, which he had observed for many years in Picardy. These observations, according to M. Bretonneau, would have contributed essentially towards a right understanding of the several mooted points, had not the writer confounded scarlatinal with diphtheritic angina.

Huxham[1] describes an epidemic in 1757, prevailing in England, which was also closely allied with scarlatina. He says:—

"Most commonly the angina came on before the exanthem, but many times the eruption appeared before the sore throat, and was sometimes very considerable, though there was little or no pain in the fauces; on the contrary, a very severe angina seized some patients that had no manner of eruption; and yet even in these cases a very great itching and desquamation sometimes ensued, but this was chiefly in grown persons, very rarely in children."

[1] Huxham, Dissertation on the Malignant Ulcerous Sore Throat. London, 1757.

The eruption was sometimes pustular, sometimes erysipelatous. He alludes to some cases in which there were signs of croup, but the symptoms were not well marked; the peculiar breathing and suffocation were wanting. He remarks that "in all sorts of fevers about this time there was a surprising disposition to eruptions of some kind or other, to soreness of throat, and apnœa." His attention was chiefly directed to the condition of the fauces, and he does not at all seem to appreciate the tendency of the disease to extend to the air-passages. Yet, by his own statements, some of his cases must have terminated with laryngeal symptoms.

"Not only," says he, "were the nostrils, fauces, &c., affected, but the windpipe itself was much corroded, and pieces of its internal membrane were spit up."

Dr. Starr, of Liskeard, published a paper in the *Philosophical Transactions*, upon the malignant ulcerous sore throat epidemic which appeared in that place in 1749. In this paper, besides other details of the epidemic, he gives 'the full data of a case in which the false membrane, commencing in the fauces, extended to the larynx. He particularly dwells upon the physical properties of the exudation, its adherence to the subjacent surface, its frequent detachment and reproduction. In fact, he gives a complete picture of Bretonneau's diphtheria.

In 1761, Rosen gives an account of an epidemic which prevailed in Sweden.

3

Dr. Samuel Bard[1] published a dissertation upon the nature, causes, and treatment of suffocative angina, as it appeared in New York in 1771. To this writer we shall have occasion to revert more particularly when we come to trace the history of diphtheria in our own country. From this period the disease and the writings which the subject had called forth, seem to have been laid aside, and almost lost sight of, when, in 1826, the treatise of Bretonneau made its appearance. This we may truly consider the first connected and practical research upon the nature of the affection. Of late, the disease has become firmly established in France, and it would seem, judging from the experience of the last few years, that it has also prevailed, to a greater or less extent, in England and in our own land. It has been described by many French writers, among whom we may mention Guersant, Isambert, Chomel, Andral, Rilliet, Barthez, Trousseau, and Bouchut.

It is by a careful study of the most characteristic and important researches into these epidemics that we are enabled to gain at least a partial insight into the nature of the disease, and to contrast the present with the earlier accounts of its character.

The epidemic at Tours, in 1818—1821, so vividly described by Bretonneau, first broke out in the barracks, amongst the soldiers, and thence spread to the surrounding quarters. Among the military the gums were the

---

[1] Researches on the Nature, Causes, and Treatment of Suffocative Angina, &c. By Samuel Bard, M. D. New York.

portions most frequently attacked, the air-passages being rarely affected. As it spread into the city, the larynx, however, was the portion which the disease selected, while the gums were unaffected; children being, in most cases, the victims.

Those who were thus attacked rarely complained much at the outset of the attack, although deglutition was slightly interfered with. On examination of the throat it was found to be somewhat inflamed; shortly a yellow-grayish patch could be seen upon the tonsils, which spread rapidly over the soft palate, the mouth, and the pharynx; the cervical and submaxillary glands became swollen and inflamed. The outward appearance of the patient, the leaden aspect, the dulness of the eye, the uncertain step, bore evidence of the severe character of the disease, while the hoarseness of the cough, the change in the tone of the voice, the extremely fetid breath, and the grayish-black exudation upon the pharynx, were speedily followed by suffocating dyspnœa and death.

From Tours the epidemic spread to two small hamlets, La Fevriere and Chanusson, to which places it was for a time confined.

"From this time it continued to traverse the departments of France, passing mainly from the southern littoral districts towards the centre. It did not seem possible to ascribe its visitations to any particular

[1] See cases reported by Bretonneau in his Treatise, 1826.

climate or meteorological conditions; for historical documents show that while it raged with terrible violence amongst the towns and hamlets of the Loiret, remarkable for their salubrity and the advantages of their geographical position, it passed over the villages of Sologne, seated amidst marshes; while elsewhere it seemed to select marshy and ill-drained districts, and to spare those which were in a better sanitary condition. Again, while in the year 1825, a year remarkable for its extreme dryness, the communes north of Orleans were laid waste by diphtheria, it made as many victims in the damp and warm year 1828, in the country south of Orleans."[1]

In this year Trousseau saw thirteen out of seventeen individuals die in the same farm-house, all attacked with diphtheria.

In 1841 an epidemic occurred in the Children's Hospital at Paris, which has been described by M. Becquerel.[2] In this many of the children were attacked with sore throat, sometimes false membranes being produced, and at others sloughs and gangrene, the one running into the other. The pharynx, larynx, and blistered surfaces were the parts attacked. In all the cases there was a want of coagulability in the blood, and pulmonary apoplexy often accompanied the malady.

In the *Archives Générales de Médecine*, M. Empis[3] gives a most valuable paper upon an epidemic of diph-

---

[1] Report of the Lancet Sanitary Commission, 1859.
[2] Gazette Médicale de Paris, 1843.   [3] March, 1850.

theria which occurred at the Hôpital Nachez, in 1848. Both the mucous and cutaneous surfaces were attacked, in many cases conjointly.

There was a very virulent epidemic in Paris in 1855, attacking the rich and poor indiscriminately; carrying off adults, but expending itself more particularly upon children.

From the early part of 1855 to March, 1857, a serious epidemic prevailed in Boulogne, during which 300 persons died, of whom many were English. A greater portion of those who were carried off were under ten years of age.

M. Lemoine has described an epidemic at Nièvre, in which the air-passages generally escaped.

In the department of the Haute Marne, the diphtheria had a decided predilection for the nasal fossæ, the larynx, for the most part, escaping. This epidemic was described by M. Jobert. M. Lespiau has given an account of an epidemic which occurred among the military-at Avignon, in the autumn of 1858, and in which the false membrane usually spread to the air-passages. Of 1796 soldiers, 195 were attacked; and of 22 children belonging to one regiment, 4 suffered. In the cases secondary to other diseases nearly all died, while in the primary cases only 6 per cent. died.

Such is a concise history of the epidemics of malignant angina which have been observed in Europe, and more especially in France, during the present century. Before giving an account of the history of diphtheria in

England, let us compare more closely the experience of French practitioners during the epidemics of the last few years with the observations of Bretonneau. We shall confine ourselves to a few of the most important points.

In his *Traité de la Diphthérite*, Bretonneau says little of the constitutional symptoms which accompany diphtheria, probably because he did not attribute to them anything more than a secondary importance. He says:—

"At the onset of diphtheria, the organic functions and those which belong to the life of relation, are so little disturbed that children who are already dangerously affected by malignant angina, generally retain their habitual appetite, and continue their play. . . . . . The disease only becomes mortal when the membranous layers which line the interior of the air-passages, form, by their accumulation, or by their adherence, a mechanical obstacle to respiration. . . . . If a topical treatment modifies the diphtheritic inflammation, the return to health follows immediately on the cessation of the local disease."[1]

In a recent paper in the *Archives Générales de Médecine*, to which we have before alluded, Bretonneau has somewhat modified his idea that diphtheria is essentially a local disease. In the recent epidemics in France, the disease has come on insidiously, and hastened to a

---

[1] Addition supplémentaire au Traité de la Diphthérite.

fatal termination in a manner not to be explained by such a theory. Still maintaining the opinion that the constitutional state of diphtheria is secondary, and incapable of existing independently of the local changes, he assumes that whenever the disease takes on a suddenly fatal form, whenever the constitutional seem to precede the local symptoms, an explanation is to be found "not in the antecedence of a morbid diathesis, but in the secret development of diphtheria in the nostrils." And this assumption seems to be founded solely upon the fact that in some cases coryza and glandular swellings have preceded the graver symptoms.

Although we cannot by any means agree with the distinguished observer in views which are so much at variance with modern experience, we must do him the justice to say that the characters of the disease, as observed by him in 1826, were undoubtedly as he has described them, but that, during the last few years, the disease has assumed new forms and been attended with new dangers. Trousseau has most distinctly admitted this change of type of diphtheria, in the *Gazette des Hôpitaux*, 1855 :—

"There is a form of diphtheria to which, for seven or eight years past, innumerable victims have succumbed, which differs so completely from all others in the general aspect of its symptoms, that one would be tempted to establish a line of demarcation; but in directing our attention to its mode of invasion and etiology, we have no difficulty in recognizing conformity and even identity; the difference being that the diphtheritic disease assumes a character of exceptional gravity, and kills at once by the constitutional affection without the participation of the larynx. Usually the sore throat seems to be the first symptom; but sometimes it is preceded by a coryza of great severity, as if the pituitary membrane had been attacked before the fauces."

"There is also swelling of the lymphatic ganglia of the neck, which is sometimes so enormous as to extend beyond the jaw.

"Join to this acute pain in the head, extremely intense fever (excessive frequency of the pulse), and you will have the signs of the onset of the worst forms of diphtheria. Some hours after you will observe false membrane on the uvula and velum; the discharge from the nose becomes fetid, and if you open the nares with an ear speculum, false membranes are observed on the septum and turbinated bones. The patient does not sleep, and is in a state of extreme agitation; the breathing is stertorous and snoring. . . . .

"After thirty-six or forty-eight hours, the features assume a livid pallor, delirium follows, and the unfortunate patient dies with all the appearance of anæmia, and in a state of somnolent tranquillity which strongly contrasts with the agitation that distinguishes the agony of croup. It is impossible to describe the horrible prostration, the powerless exhaustion, the frequent faintings, in one of which the thread of life is often severed."

Again, in the course of a report read before the

Imperial Academy of Medicine, on the 2d November, 1851, M. Trousseau makes the following remarks:—

"Those of us who for twenty-five years have followed the epidemics of diphtheria which have stricken the capital, may satisfy ourselves that the disease has not only extended itself considerably, particularly during the last twelve or thirteen years, but has assumed a much graver form. Up to about 1846, diphtheria scarcely appeared in the epidemic form, and the cases of it which were observed in Paris presented all the characters so well described by Bretonneau in his treatise, and so clearly pointed out by Guersant in the *Dictionnaire de Médecine*, where this excellent practitioner confirms in every particular what the illustrious physician of Tours had seen. . . . .

"The diphtherite described by Bretonneau generally commenced in the pharynx, and there remained the longer in proportion to the youth of the child, giving rise usually to but little fever, scarcely in any way affecting the rest of the economy, and was propagated to the larynx, thus constituting croup. But within the last ten years, in place of this affection, comparatively of little severity, there has appeared another, in which hitherto all the resources of art have been nearly unavailing.

"The pharynx, it is true, is most commonly first attacked, but in a little time the disease extends to the nares, to the nasal duct, and sometimes to the internal surface of the eyelids; and at the same time ataxoadynamic symptoms become manifest, the pulse becomes very frequent, the cervical glands greatly enlarge, and frequently forty-eight hours after the attack, the patient dies, *without the larynx having been sufficiently affected to suggest the idea of croup.* It seems as though a poison had been introduced into the system, by which the latter had been intimately and rapidly modified."

So also in the account given by M. Isambert[1] of the epidemic in Paris in 1856, we find, under the head of malignant diphtheritic angina, the following observations:—

"We retain the old name of malignant angina to designate that specific form in which the patient succumbs to a profound adynamia, to a general intoxication, and in nowise to the occlusion of the larynx. For in cases of this description tracheotomy not only does not save, but it does not even temporarily relieve the patient. This form of angina seems to have escaped the notice of M. Bretonneau, and as we cannot suppose that a man of his powers of observation could overlook a type of the disease so well marked, we must admit that it did not present itself in those epidemics, in the midst of which the eminent physician wrote his *Traité de la Diphthérite.* This form, then, appears to be a new one, although without doubt it is to this that many of the descriptions of the malignant or gangrenous anginas of the early epidemics apply."

---

[1] Arch. Gén. de Médecine, 1857.

Having described the anatomical lesions, the enormous tumefaction of the cervical glands, and the other local changes, he goes on to say:—

"These local disorders, so grave in character, are accompanied by a general state not less serious: burning fever, extreme restlessness, insupportable headache, depriving the patient of all sleep, are present; shortly typhoid symptoms, the most complete adynamia, declare themselves; the fever appears to diminish towards the end, the pulse becomes small, and the patient falls into a condition of somnolent tranquillity, which announces the termination."

Were it necessary, in order to prove that the constitutional symptoms of diphtheria have not only been present, but have often assumed a primary importance during the epidemics of the last few years, we might refer to many other papers published by French practitioners. We shall have occasion to observe the importance of these symptoms when we study the history of the English epidemics.

One of the points most particularly insisted upon by M. Bretonneau is the absence of all relation between diphtheria and gangrene of the fauces. He even considers it characteristic of the affection that the mucous membrane remains unaltered throughout. He says that malignant angina is unaccompanied with any sloughing, and a contrary opinion could only arise from deceptive appearances, for in none of the cases at Tours, even when malignant angina had assumed the most repulsive aspect, could anything be discovered which resembled a gangrenous lesion.

In this opinion he certainly seems to be supported by historical testimony, especially as regards some of the epidemics of the last century.

"The results of the analysis of historical testimony do not differ in any respect from those which my own direct observations furnish me."[1] But in others of the recent French epidemics, in which researches were conducted with a special view to a solution of this point, gangrene has occurred as the expected termination of all the most malignant cases, and not as a mere accident. In the epidemic at Paris in 1841, described by M. Becquerel, and to which we have already referred, gangrenous sore throat prevailed at the same time with cases which presented the true characters of diphtheria. The two forms of disease were not to be distinguished as respects their origin, the local affection not being preceded by any constitutional symptoms. The fauces, too, in all cases, at first presented appearances purely diphtheritic. In those which in their progress took on the gangrenous aspect, the exudation became friable, and soon separated from the mucous surface. At first this was usually entire, but exhibited the appearance of a limited eschar, and, on being thrown off, left a deep excavation. The constitutional symptoms preceding death were the same as those

---

[1] Traité de la Diphthérite, p. 13.

which usually accompany gangrene—diminution of tem·
perature, a rapid and almost imperceptible pulse, great
restlessness, frequent vomiting, involuntary stools, &c.
These cases were generally fatal.

From the fact that many of these cases were examined
after death, there is no reason to suppose that there
could be any mistake as to the actual presence of gangrene. In 15 cases examined, there was gangrene affecting the tonsils exclusively in 9, and in the remaining 6,
the pillars of the velum and pharynx. In the tonsil, the
gangrene was either in the centre or near the surface.
In either case, the resulting cavity was irregular in form,
filled with a thin fetid fluid, and was surrounded by
softening of the submucous tissue, which was to a
greater or less extent converted into greenish-gray
detritus. The disintegration evidently commenced beneath the mucous membrane, which, at first merely
swollen and rugose, gradually took on a gangrenous
appearance and color, and finally terminated in an
eschar. When this separated, the cavity was left
exposed.

The history of this epidemic clearly shows that
although the gangrenous form of diphtheria differs from
the purely membranous in various ways, yet it occurs
under the same epidemic influence.

M. Isambert, in his account of the Paris epidemics of
1855 and '56, distinguishes both forms of diphtheria, the
one tending to a fatal result by extension to the larynx,

4

the other, which he calls angina maligna diphtheritica, assuming a totally different character.

"It is particularly to this form," he says, "that are to be referred those confluent exudations of a dirty gray or black color, giving out a gangrenous odor. . . . Several times we have observed undoubted loss of substance beneath the exudation."[1]

Again:—

"In this disease the membranous exudation, soon after its appearance, softens, and assumes a dirty gray or blackish color, the uncovered mucous surface is livid, the adenetic swelling is enormous, and affects not only the glands themselves, but the cellular tissue, the skin often sloughing from extensive tension."

Death is preceded by gradually increasing prostration, but not accompanied by any nervous symptoms more marked than those described by M. Becquerel in the account of his epidemic.

M. Duche gives a description of the diphtherite which has proved so fatal for the last few years in the department of L'Yonne.

"The principal features of this epidemic (1858) are cephalalgia, fever more or less intense, and pain in the fauces. Upon examining the mouth, the tonsils are found swollen and red, and on the surface of one—sometimes on both at the same time—there is a white patch of variable dimensions. These patches quickly enlarge,

[1] Archives Générales, 1857.

reach the velum palati and uvula, which latter, at times, becomes enormously enlarged; later, they invade the posterior wall of the pharynx, and descend gradually into the larynx and bronchia, and even into the œsophagus and digestive organs.

"The first period, which may be called pharyngeal, is characterized by a painful sensation, and the ejection from the mouth of abundant sputa, mixed with blood and false membrane. The invasion of the larynx is marked by all the signs of croup, and asphyxia rapidly terminates the scene of agony. On the contrary, when the larynx escapes, there is an apparent calm, which deceives the most experienced eyes. Then there is a little vomiting of glairy matter, great thirst, absence of pain, but, soon complete prostration; pulse insensible; absence of urine during four or five days, and death by syncope.

"It is generally easy, by aid of curved forceps, to seize and tear away the membranous exudations, when they cover only the tonsils, uvula, or pharynx. The mucous membrane, thus denuded, is livid and bloody; and in spite of the most energetic cauterizations, a few hours suffice for the reappearance of new morbid formations like the first. Gangrene of the pharynx often terminates the disease in a sudden manner, and we are warned of this fatal issue by the fetor of the breath, and of substances ejected from the mouth."

According to Bretonneau, diphtheria also includes croup. He says: "Croup is but the extreme degree of malignant angina." Now, it would certainly seem very evident, to those of us who have derived our ideas of the word croup from Dr. Francis Home's description of this affection,[1] or from the graphic lecture on Cynanche trachealis, by Dr. Watson, that Bretonneau uses the word in a very different sense.

It is well known that Dr. Home first introduced the term croup into medical literature in 1765, and to him is due the honor of first defining the characters of a disease which had been in part described by the most ancient authors. He first drew attention to the fact, that the formation of a false membrane in the trachea and larynx is essential to the disease, and constitutes the source of danger.

Dr. Home's description of croup was not only accepted by most of the physicians of England, but also by many in Europe. His views were especially supported by the writings of Cheyne, Cullen, and others, but still more particularly by the report of the commissioners of the famous *concours* instituted by Napoleon. The ideas of these writers were, in brief—

"That croup is an acute inflammation of the mucous membrane of the air-passages, distinguished from others by the rapidity of its progress; by the existence of concrete exudation in the larynx, and by the fact that it principally attacks children under ten years of age. They regard cold and moisture as its main causes, and support this inference by all that is known as to the

---

[1] Inquiry into the Nature, Cause, and Cure of the Croup—Edinboro', 1765.

seasons during which the disease is most apt to occur,
and the climates in which it is most prevalent; and they
hold that it is its habit, to select for its invasion, single
individuals in large populations, without communicating
itself to the rest—in other words, that it is apt to be
sporadic, not epidemic."

Dr. Watson, in his lectures, says:—

"Some analogy with that disease (croup) it certainly
has, but the points of difference are stronger and more
essential. It resembles croup, inasmuch as it leads to
the production of an adventitious membrane upon a
mucous surface. It differs in the position of that membrane, which is seldom formed in the trachea. The
affection of the windpipe, when it occurs at all, is secondary, so that the term 'cynanche trachealis' would be
quite inappropriate."

In an admirable lecture on Diphtheria, by Dr.
Ranking, and published in the *Lancet*,[1] we find the
following remarks:—

"The great distinctive mark between diphtherite and
croup, properly so called, is to be found in the locality
chiefly affected. In both, it is true, a main feature is the
presence of an exudation; but in the one disease, it
commences in the fauces, and only reaches the windpipe
by extension, and in a certain number of cases; in the
other, that of true croup: it commences in the larynx
and trachea, and does not necessarily affect the soft parts
above the glottis at all. As a consequence of this, a

[1] The Lancet, Jan. 15, 1859.

marked difference is also found in the symptoms of the two diseases. In diphtheria the uneasiness is first referred to the parts subservient to deglutition; in croup, on the contrary, the earliest symptom is that of stridulous voice and breathing—a symptom which, in the former, indicates the final development of diseased action."

Dr. Hauner,[1] director of the children's hospital at Munich, concludes a paper upon this subject with the following aphorisms:—

"1. True croup (laryngeal croup) is a disease proper to childhood, and its cause is chiefly to be sought in the organization (the period of development) of the larynx at this period of life. 2. The anatomy and physiology of the larynx sufficiently explain the nature of croup. 3. It cannot be shown that croup is connected with any peculiarity of the blood crasis. 4. True croup always commences in the larynx, and often passes downwards to the trachea, &c., but it never passes upwards. 5. Laryngeal croup is characterized by a pseudo-membrane of more or less extent. 6. Laryngeal croup is to be carefully distinguished from diphtheritic croup, the latter always depending upon a peculiar blood crasis, as seen in other organs of enfeebled individuals. 7. Diphtheritic croup is almost always secondary, and is not essentially different from croup in an after acute exanthemata. 8. The diphtheritic form begins, as a general rule, in the fauces, uvula, tonsils, &c., and

[1] Journal für Kinderkrankheiten.

extends hence downwards. It is very rare for it to commence in the larynx or trachea, &c."

It is well known that Dr. West, in his work upon diseases of children, has considered diphtheritis as a form of croup. In the last edition of his work, however, he has seen fit to modify his previous views. In speaking of croup and diphtheria, he says:—

"Of these two diseases, the one is almost always idiopathic, the other is often secondary; the one attacks persons in perfect health, is sthenic in its character, acute in its course, and usually proves amenable to antiphlogistic treatment. The other attacks by preference those who are out of health, or who are surrounded by unfavorable hygienic conditions, and is remarkable for the asthenic character of the symptoms which attend it. The one selects its victims almost exclusively from among children; is incapable of being diffused by contagion; is governed in its prevalence by influence of season, temperature, and climate, but rarely becomes, in the usual acceptation of the term, an epidemic. While the other attacks adults as well as children, is propagated by contagion, and, though it occasionally occurs in a sporadic form, is susceptible of wide-spread epidemic influence.

. . . . "Different, however, as are the two diseases, there are yet between them points of similarity no less striking, and the diagnostic difficulties are still further enhanced by the occasional simultaneous prevalence of both affections.

. . . . "It has, indeed, been suggested by M. Lam-
bert, in a recent valuable paper, that the condition of
the subjacent mucous membrane furnishes a ground of
distinction between the affections; and that while in
diphtheria the surface beneath the exudation is often
ulcerated, no such erosion of the mucous membrane is
met with in true croup. This is not, however, according to my observation, for ulceration of the mucous
membrane has come under my notice in primary croup,
though less frequently than in cases of the diphtheritic
kind.

"Whatever differences exist between croup and diphtheria, must be sought elsewhere than in the pathological changes observable in the respiratory organs;
and the affinities of the latter disease are seen to be to
the class of blood diseases, rather than to that of purely
local inflammation to which croup belongs."

With Bretonneau, nearly all French writers regard
croup and diphtheria as identical. In justification of
this view, so little consonant with our own ideas, we
may remark that in France, true croup is commonly
introduced by a diphtheritic affection of the fauces, and
that sometimes it appears to be contagious, which is not
considered to be true of the sporadic disease as observed
in England and in our country. Moreover, in France,
it differs by its asthenic character, and to some extent
by the nature of the exudation, which is less tenacious.

In fine, the laryngeal diphtheritis of Bretonneau, and
of other French authors, although closely resembling

the disease described by Home, and known to us as croup in its anatomical characters, differs widely in its dynamical ones. Moreover, it is contagious and epidemic.

Bretonneau has also in a measure confounded scarlatina with diphtheria under the term "Scarlatina Anginosa."

The exact relation which exists between these two diseases has been a much debated question. By some persons the two affections, notwithstanding certain points of strong resemblance, are regarded as essentially different. By others, diphtheria is looked upon as a form of scarlet fever, in which the throat affection is unaccompanied by the eruption which usually characterizes it.

We must admit that there are many circumstances which favor this latter opinion. For instance, not only do the two diseases prevail frequently at the same time in the same region, but even in the same family; some members being attacked by all the symptoms of true diphtheria, while others present the symptoms of common scarlatina. Then, again, in some instances, in those who have been attacked by diphtheria, a rash very similar to that of scarlatina has been observed. This rash may have been very partial, and may have remained but a few hours, but its characters have been thought sufficiently marked to leave no doubt as to its nature. Moreover, since the albuminous condition of the urine has been so frequently observed in cases of diphtheria, it may be thought that the analogy between the two diseases is drawn still closer.

These facts are certainly of great weight, but we shall see that there are other considerations still stronger which may be adduced in favor of the essential difference between the two diseases. For example, as regards the existence of a rash. This has certainly been occasionally noticed in some epidemics of diphtheria, but in the great majority it has not been observed at all. Whereas, in epidemics of scarlet fever its absence is a rare exception, and occurs only in those cases of very malignant character which are marked by great cerebral disturbance, violent delirium, and by speedy death. In diphtheria, on the other hand, the intellect remains undisturbed until the very last.

Then, again, the rash is in many respects dissimilar from that seen in scarlatina. It is described as being for the most part, of a uniform erythematous redness, without the peculiar punctated appearance of the scarlet fever rash, appearing suddenly in patches, not deepening in intensity gradually, and not followed by any change in the other symptoms, nor by any increase in their severity.

As to the presence of albumen in the urine, there are certain points to be especially observed. When present there is no diminution in the quantity of the secretion, neither is there any other particular change in its character. Moreover, the albumen seems often to disappear at a very early period of the disease.

"Its disappearance takes place suddenly, and though its presence is usually observed in cases where this disease is severe, yet there does not seem to be any necessary connection between the urine becoming non-albuminous, and the disease assuming a milder type."

Again, the sequelæ of the two diseases are widely different. For while, on the one hand, we have none of the formidable dropsical symptoms in the convalescence of diphtheria, which so often succeed scarlatina, on the other, we *do* have a peculiar loss of nervous power, and temporary muscular paralysis which have no analogy to anything in the sequelæ of the latter disease.

Dr. Greenhow, in his excellent monograph[1] on this disease, says:—

"Besides the absence after diphtheria of the well known sequelæ of scarlet fever, the former disease is succeeded by sequelæ of a character peculiar to itself, and such as have not been found to follow scarlet fever. These are partial paralysis of the muscles of deglutition and voice, impairment or disorder of vision, paraplegia, hemiplegia, partial paralysis of the upper extremities, numbness of the hands or feet, tenderness, pricking or tingling of the extremities, and gastrodynia. Then, lastly, the occurrence of diphtheria on other parts of the body, as on abrasions of the skin or wounds, or on the pudenda, has no parallel in scarlet fever. When to these differences we add that the anæmia which soon

[1] On Diphtheria, by Edw. Headlam Greenhow, M. D., F. R. C. P. N. Y., 1861.

occurs, and for a long time succeeds to diphtheria, is more intense than in almost any other acute disease, there can be little hesitation in accepting the conclusion that diphtheria and scarlet fever are not the same disease."

Lastly, almost universal experience bears testimony to this fact, viz., that diphtheria does not protect from scarlet fever, nor, on the other hand, does scarlet fever prove any defence against diphtheria. Of this the following may serve as examples:—

"Three children in a family in my district (Islington) were attacked with diphtheria in August, 1858. Two of them died; the third, aged three years, recovered. I saw these children, and satisfied myself that there was no error in the diagnosis. In January, 1859, the child that recovered was attacked with scarlet fever, after playing about upon a carpet brought from a house where a fatal case of this disease had occurred. There was both the rash, and the usual throat affection, but no diphtheritic exudation; and the child died."[1]

Dr. West gives the following case:—

"In a school in the neighborhood of London, diphtheria broke out; many of the lads were affected by it, and one or two died. Several of those who were convalescent from the disease were sent to the sea coast for the more speedy recovery of their strength, and while there some were attacked by scarlet fever, and this also, in one or two cases, proved fatal."[2]

---

[1] Dr. Edw. Ballard, Med. Times and Gazette, July 23, 1859.
[2] Dr. West, Diseases of Childhood, 1859.

Dr. Greenhow states that, at the outset of his inquiries, he was inclined to doubt that diphtheria was entirely distinct from scarlatina. But careful observation and more ample experience have satisfied him that notwithstanding their frequent occurrence in the same place, and their occasional coincidence in the same individual, diphtheria and scarlatina are distinct diseases.

Numerous cases similar to these might be cited. And, although further and more accurate observations may hereafter tend to a different conclusion, we are decidedly of the opinion that the balance of evidence at the present time is in favor of the non-identity of scarlatina and diphtheria.

As regards the history of the earlier epidemics of "sore throat" in England, we have few reliable accounts, and even of the origin and progress of the late epidemics of diphtheria, our knowledge is far from being either accurate or satisfactory. We have already alluded to the description of the epidemics of throat disease by Fothergill and Huxham, about the middle of the last century, as also to the admirable paper of Dr. Starr. The first of these writers, as we have seen, speaks distinctly of sloughs in the fauces which leave ulcers. Huxham and Starr speak of the exudation extending to the air-passages. It is not a little remarkable, that the same neighborhood in Cornwall (Liskeard and the other towns in which the epidemic of ulcerous sore throat described by Dr. Huxham prevailed), has been subject

5

during the last three years to a similar affection, and which closely resembles the disease described by M. Becquerel, inasmuch as the membranous exudation of unusual thickness is associated with softening and destruction of the submucous tissue. This epidemic has been well described by Mr. Thompson, of Launceston.[1]

"About three years since, this neighborhood was visited by an epidemic of this disease. The first cases occurred in the town; and no others then appeared for several months, when it again broke out in the district north of this place, where it prevailed for several months; whilst the south side was comparatively free from it. From the north it gradually spread until the whole line of country had been visited by it. There appeared to be no difference in the geological nature of the country, the level, or the aspect, in increasing the severity, or granting an immunity from the disease. The premonitory symptoms varied somewhat. A few retired to rest comparatively well, and awoke in the morning with the throat sore, and covered with white deposit. In the majority it was preceded by all the ordinary symptoms of pyrexia, of which headache was one of the most severe; followed in the course of a day or two by the usual throat symptoms. An extreme feeling of depression, not to be accounted for by the amount of mischief in the throat, was a characteristic

[1] Brit. Med. Journal, June, 1858.

symptom in each case. An external examination of the throat showed the tonsil generally to be swollen, hard, and tender to the touch; whilst sometimes the parotid gland participated in the swelling. Internally the tonsil was swollen, and either covered with the diphtheritic deposit which frequently extended over the pharynx, and sometimes into the nares and palate; or else it would be scooped out into an ulcer with raised violet-colored edges; the floor exhibiting a dark ash-colored slough. In some instances there would be no deposit or ulceration at first, but simply the tonsil painful and enlarged. These cases generally change for a state of ulceration, which began in several distinct spots, and gradually spread over the whole tonsil. In the most severe examples, the tonsil sometimes sloughed *en masse*. I saw one instance in which this occurred in an early stage of the disease, and where now (two years since it occurred) a cavity remains capable of containing a pigeon's egg, across the surface of which extends a small band of mucous membrane which did not slough at the same time, and gives great inconvenience from retaining the food impacted in the hollow during deglutition. I have seen no case in which I could detect the extension of the disease into the œsophagus; but in many it has entered into the air-passages, this being the most frequent and most fatal complication."

"It can scarcely fail to strike the reader that the affection under consideration would be just as correctly designated by the term 'sore throat with ulcers,' employed by Huxham and Fothergill, as by that of diphtheria, a fact which appears the more remarkable when we consider that the very towns in which Huxham's disease most prevailed in 1748–50, have been most severely visited during the last few years. Are these two epidemics, separated by an interval of more than a century, of the same nature? A careful comparison of their symptoms assures us that they are, and that Bretonneau, in disclaiming all relationship between his diphtheria and the 'sore throat with ulcers,' was mistaken."[1]

As we have before remarked, in the year 1765 Dr. Home published a small treatise[2] upon a disease of the larynx which had long been known, but the characters of which had never been clearly defined. To this he gave the name of croup, and upon this essay the modern doctrine of croup is based. Home's description is based upon the careful observation of twelve cases, in ten of which post-mortem examinations were made. He first pointed out that the formation of a false membrane is essential to the disease, and that its presence in the larynx is the source of danger. Others also published their observations upon this disease, among whom were Cheyne and Cullen. The affection described by these writers is essentially different from the croup of Bretonneau.

---

[1] Brit. and For. Med.-Chir. Review, Jan. 1860.
[2] Inquiry into the Nature, Cause, and Cure of Croup, Edinb., 1765.

From this time, until its recent outbreak, although we may gather a few scattering allusions to diphtheria from British medical literature, it was a disease practically unknown to even the most experienced of English practitioners, certainly, in the form in which it has of late presented itself.

The advent of the present epidemics of the disease attracted public attention in England, in the autumn of 1857, a few cases having occurred for twelve months previously. It first appeared in the southeastern counties, especially in Kent, in the town of Canterbury. In Essex, particularly in the marshy districts, it prevailed extensively; thence it spread through all the eastern counties.

"The local name was 'throat fever.' It appeared after arriving at a certain stage to baffle medical skill, and something of a fungus nature showed itself in the throat. Croupal suffocation was one of its complications, which appears to eliminate 'putrid sore throat,' and those, therefore, who classify this Cornish epidemic with diphtheria are probably warranted in so doing."[1]

During the next summer months the disease spread northwards to Lincolnshire and Yorkshire. In the winter months of 1858 the southeastern counties still suffered. In parts of Essex the disease was almost universal.

[1] On Diphtheria, by Ernest Hart, London, 1859.

"At Teignmouth, Mr. Lake observed cases of that severest form of diphtheric inflammation, in which the local manifestation of the disease is from the first overshadowed in importance by the constitutional symptoms. The blood-making powers were seriously compromised after the annihilation of the throat affection, the patient sinking then through general failure of the powers of life, without anything like typhoid symptoms, a distinction which it is very important to maintain, or being left in a state in which he is liable to be carried off by any prevalent disorder, or during convalescence continuing unusually weak and anæmic."

In Suffolk, and in some of the eastern counties, as also in Nottinghamshire, scarlatina prevailed in conjunction with diphtheria. In the northwestern counties we find hooping-cough and diphtheria prevailing.

In fact the disease spread to almost all parts of England, appearing with much greater severity in some localities than in others. Dr. Hart has given in his report a very succinct account of its progress through the country.

If now we examine some of the various accounts of the recent epidemics in England, as they have appeared in different parts of the country, there will be seen to be a considerable amount of discrepance, and, moreover, many of the accounts will be found to differ widely from Bretonneau's model. We select a few as they have appeared in the various journals of the day :—

At a meeting of the Harveian Society,[1] Dr. B. Sanderson said :—

"That the disease recently prevalent in England was identical with the malignant sore throat described by many authors, and that in a great number of instances scarlatina precedes it. It was attended with much fever and fetid breath, the fever sometimes of a typhoid character. The thickness and adhesiveness of the exudation were less marked than that occurring at Tours. In England exhaustion and fever destroyed the patient rather than asphyxia, which suddenly put an end to Bretonneau's patients. In true diphtheria there was no fever and no fetid breath; both these were remarked in this country. Finally, he believed croup and diphtheria identical, and that the disease in England was not diphtherite, but the pultaceous pharyngitis of the French."

Dr. Laycock, of Edinburgh, in a clinical lecture, published in May, 1858, regards diphtheria as a disease produced by a fungous growth—"oïdium albicans"—similar to that found in thrush. He says :—

"If the fungus multiply in a population at the same time that there is an epidemic of scarlatina or rubeola prevalent, that epidemic may be expected to take the diphtheritic form."

His remarks, however, appear to be based solely on the following case, in which there was an aphthous affection of the mouth and throat.

James D——, aged 35, married—admitted into the

Infirmary March 19—stated that, until two years ago, his health was good. About that time he had diarrhœa with frequent desire to go to stool, and much straining at stool without result. A few weeks afterwards had shiverings and sweatings, and a peculiar feeling of numbness, with loss of sensibility in upper and lower extremities. The arms would become stiff. At present, the attacks of stiffness come on only when his hands are placed behind the back. Continued at work until eight days ago.

On examination it was found that he slept well, swallowed easily, had no pain after eating, but was flatulent. Bowels regular, motions solid. Abdomen large and tumid. Urine of spec. grav. 100.5, no albumen, no sugar—amount seventy ounces per diem. Under the microscope, the blood was seen to contain colorless corpuscles in slightly increased quantity. Lungs healthy, no cough or expectoration. His skin under the clothing was pale; the inner surface of the lips pallid, the face unusually brown, but evidently from atmospheric pressure. In three weeks after admission, the bowels became relaxed, and by April 13 an obstinate diarrhœa had set in, which resisted all the usual remedies. On the 15th he complained of sore throat, and on examination, the fauces were seen to be deeply congested, and covered with white spots. The tongue had also white patches upon it. He still complained of the hyperæsthetic sensations in his arms, and was hopeless as to his recovery. On April 23, pulse 120, deglutition difficult, with a constant burning pain in the throat. On the 24th the pharynx was seen to be covered with a thick yellowish pellicle, and the surface beneath, when it was detached, was raw and bleeding. The pellicle, when a fragment was placed under the microscope, was found to consist of the mycelium and sporules of the oïdium albicans, with epithelium and pus cells. He was ordered the aqua chlorinata, and a solution to the fauces of nitrate of silver. . . . . The patient gradually sank until the morning of the 11th inst., when he died.

Autopsy.—On removing the tongue, trachea and œsophagus, it was found that a soft yellowish-white pultaceous matter was adherent to the mucous membrane of the tongue, pharynx, and œsophagus. This occurred in some places as a continuous layer, in other places as patches. It could be readily scraped off, when the mucous membrane was found to present a somewhat raw appearance. It was most abundant in the pharynx over the back of the larynx. The matter extended down the œsophagus to within two inches of the stomach. On examining microscopically the matter found on the mucous membrane, it was seen to consist of the branching filaments and sporules of the oïdium albicans, mixed with large quantities of somewhat altered epithelial scales. The larynx and trachea were quite natural. . . . . The mesentery was found to be converted into a large cancerous mass; the lumbar glands and supra-renal capsules were also implicated in the same disease.

Comment by Dr. Laycock.—The immediate cause of death was the exhausting diarrhœa. Now this supervened coincidently with an attack of diphtheria. At the onset of the disease, and just at the period before death, we found in the pellicle formed on the tongue and fauces, the sporules and mycelium of the oïdium albicans, a parasitic fungus found also in muguet, the epidemic aphtha or diphtheria of infants in France. This is an interesting fact at the present moment, when diphtherite is prevailing, more especially as the pellicle was also found abundantly after death in the œsophagus. I have little doubt that this pellicle was due to the action of the parasite on the enfeebled mucous surface of the mouth, fauces, &c. It acts like all its tribe, as an irritant inducing increased formation of epithelial scales, and effusion of mucous exudation, corpuscles or plasma; intermingled among these are the sporules, and the mycelium of the microscopic fungus; the whole constitutes a pellicle or membrane, varying in thickness. (Fig. 1.) The parasite seems to act upon the capillaries of the subjacent tissue, as, when removed, blood is not uncommonly effused, and the surface looks raw. Diphtheria is not, however, limited to one form of disease. . . . . If the fungus multiply in a population at the same time that there is an epidemic of scarlatina or rubeola prevalent therein, that epidemic may be expected to take the diphtheritic form in those cases which are attacked by the oïdium. I must add, however, that we have had reasons for thinking that the oïdium, acting alone, will fasten upon the mucous membrane of the mouth and throat, and excite inflammation and without the formation of a pellicle. . . . . The diagnosis

Fig. 1.

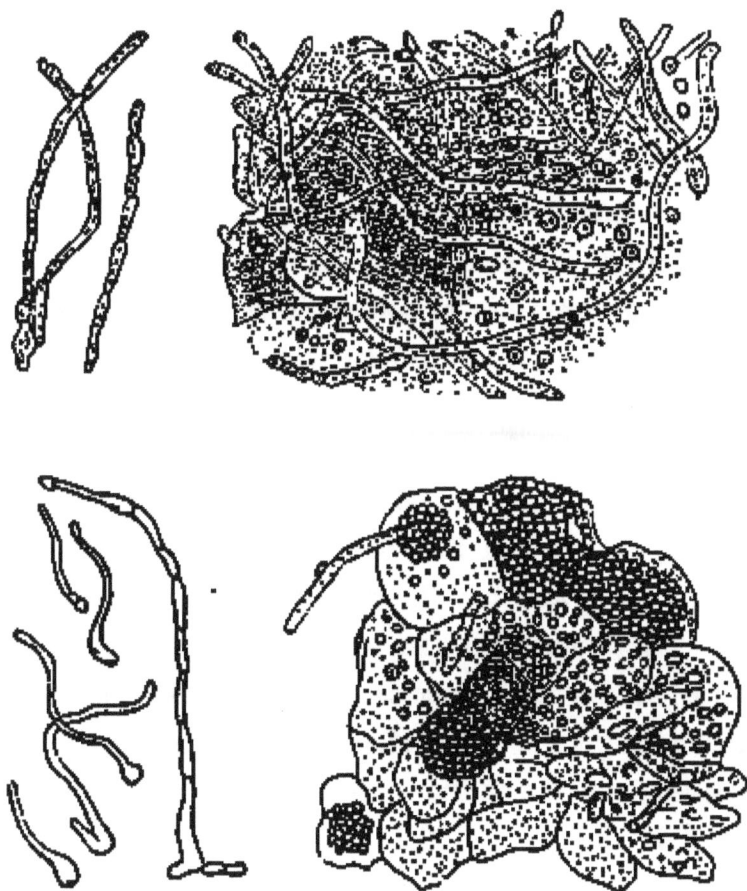

The sporules and the mycelium of the oïdium. After Robin.

of diphtheritic oïdium from ordinary aphtha is founded, first, on the character of the morbid appearance, for, in ordinary aphtha, the disease is vesicular, and the white specks or patches are ulcers, while in diphtheria, they

are pellicular, and not ulcerative, while the redness is
much deeper than in aphtha. Besides, the microscope
may reveal the spores and mycelium of the fungus. The
development of the mycelium is, however, by no means
a necessary result of the action of the fungus. This
seems to be peculiar to the more advanced stages; at
first there is not even a pellicle, only characteristic redness of the affected surface. . . . . Further, it is probable that besides the stage of development, the condition
of the *habitat* may make a considerable difference as to
the morbid products. . . . . How great a share these
microscopic parasitic organisms have in the causation of
disease, remains yet to be ascertained.

In answer to remarks made by Dr. Rogers, that he not
only thinks diphtheria to be a blood disease, but that, *as
such*, it cannot be a parasitic disease, Dr. Laycock says
(*Lancet*, Jan. 22 and 29, 1859): "Comparative pathology
teaches, however, that this conclusion is at least doubtful. The muscardine (an epizootic disease of the silk-
worm) is due to a species of fungus like that which
infects the potato, called, after its discoverer, the Botrytis
bassiana, and the sporules are described as being reproduced in the blood of the insect when it becomes acid;
while the filaments and mycelium appear on the respiratory surfaces, that is, at the outlets of the tracheal
tubes.

"Again, the fungus of the common house fly (Myco-
phyton Cohnii) is a mould or oïdium found in the blood,
abdomen, and sometimes in the intestines of the insect at

beginning of autumn. Its first symptom observed, is a milky appearance of the blood. It is found in the blood in all stages of development, from the simple minute spore or cell, to the full-grown mycelium. It is found in like manner in the fluids of the intestines, and appears externally as a mould. Flies thus affected may be often seen sticking with outstretched wings to the window panes at the end of the summer and beginning of autumn. These are by no means solitary instances of parasitic blood disease. Indeed, hamatophyta, as Lebert terms these microscopic blood parasites, infest the blood of several classes of insects. The same facts also hold good as to the vegetable parasites. . . . . These are facts which ought to make us hesitate, at least in coming to the conclusion, in the absence of all inquiry, that a parasitic disease cannot be a blood disease in man.

. . . . "That these parasites are sometimes powerful irritants of the lining tissues, is, I think, fully established both from the history of muguet and other circumstances, and although French writers speak of *pseudo-diphtherite*, the accuracy of the term may be questioned, for the exudation appears externally on ulcerated or exposed surfaces, as well as internally, in both muguet and diphtheria alike. An interesting case of vaginal blennorrhœa, due probably to oïdium albicans introduced from without, may be found in *Archiv für Physiologie*, vol. ix. p. 466. The labia were swollen, the vagina of a bright-red, studded with enlarged papillæ, and covered with star-like patches of membrane, like

6

those of the mouth in muguet, which were found to
contain the O. albicans. The patient in the next bed
had subsequently active fever, abdominal tenderness, O.
albicans of the mouth with muguet.

"It is usual to speak of the characteristic pellicle as
if it were peculiar to diphtheria, but this is by no means
the case. It is not unfrequently seen in cases of typhus
and relapsing fever, sometimes in yellow fever, and I
believe in all fevers. A series of carefully conducted
experiments, made with a thorough knowledge of
cryptogamic botany on lower animals so as to show the
real pathological origin and the effects of these parasitic
fungi, would be very valuable. . . . . . I am inclined
to think that it would probably be shown that these
parasites may act either through the blood or locally
only.

"I may observe, in conclusion, that antiseptics and
parasiticides appear to be the most efficient remedies in
diphtheria. I can speak very favorably of the tinct. of
the sesquichloride of iron (an antiseptic and hydro-
chlorate of potass)."

Dr. Kingsford,[1] in a letter to the *Lancet*, thus speaks
of the disease as it has come under his observation:—

"Diphtheria may be divided into the mild and severe
forms.

"The mild form, which, for the sake of distinction,
may be designated the diphtheritic sore throat, is ushered

in by a variable amount of feverishness, loss of appetite, and at first only slight pain in swallowing; the tongue presents a thick, white, creamy coat, through which some of the papillæ are visible; the velum palati, uvula, and pharynx are of a bright red color; the tonsils are much swollen, and of the same livid hue, and upon the inner side of one or both of them distinct white patches are seen, which in some instances resemble an exudation from the sulci of the tumid gland, but more frequently are flat and filmy in appearance, not confined to the tonsils alone, but spread over the uvula and posterior wall of the pharynx; both the exudation and the filmy deposit adhere tenaciously to the submucous surface, and cannot easily be scraped off. Ulcerative stomatitis not rarely precedes and accompanies this mild form of diphtheria—indeed, by some they are considered to be identical; the parotid and submaxillary glands are not much swollen, although one or two enlarged glandulæ concatenatæ may often be detected.

"The severe form, or genuine diphtheria, is always characterized by a high state of fever, hot, pungent skin, flushed countenance, congested lips, a rapid, feeble pulse, great difficulty in swallowing, and hurried respiration; the tongue is covered by a thick, dirty, yellowish-brown or sometimes slaty-colored coat; the velum palati, uvula and pharynx are of a deep, dark, erysipelatous redness; the tonsils usually enormously swollen, and of the same dark red color, but instead of the white patches observed in the mild form a large ash-colored membrane is spread over the inner side of one or both tonsils, and also upon the uvula and posterior wall of the pharynx. As the disease advances, the above symptoms increase in severity; the breathing becomes stertorous from mechanical obstruction; deglutition so painful that young children will refuse to swallow even liquids; the saliva dribbles from the mouth, and a foul acrid discharge often flows from the nares; the pulse becomes more rapid and feeble; the glands of the neck are now swollen and tender, and the voice is hoarse and indistinct; the patient restless, tosses about upon the bed, or else lies on his back in a semi-comatose state. These cases, when fatal, terminate either by rapid prostration of the vital powers, or by an affection simulating croup, from extension of the diphtheritic membrane into the air-passages; in both instances death is usually preceded by obstinate vomiting, probably the result of inflammation or irritation of the par vagum. . . .

"In fatal cases, the *post-mortem* examination reveals the ash-colored membrane spread over the pharynx, extending to the posterior nares and down the œsophagus; but when death is preceded by symptoms of croup, it is found also in the larynx and trachea. Upon detaching this membranous exudation, the submucous surface presents an ecchymosed appearance, but no distinct signs of ulceration."

Dr. Heslop, in a communication to the *Medical Times and Gazette*,[1] expresses his belief that, although so little

---

[1] May 29, 1858.

known now, this disease was well understood and described by former British authors, especially Fothergill.
It is a pestilence with well-marked features. It is contagious, though not highly so, and its ataxic phenomena
are most striking—prostration, quite disproportionate to
the amount of disease in the throat, coming on early,
and remaining after all other indications of disease have
passed away. In the worst cases a foul, ulcerous condition of the fauces complicates the genuine membranous
angina. The mode of death, as in other pestilences, is
by asthenia, and frequently the event is sudden and un-
looked for.

Dr. Heslop points out in detail the differences between
this affection and croup.

Dr. Whitehead, in the same journal, describing the
disease, states that the symptoms are very similar to
those of croup, but that they come on suddenly, without
the peculiar crowing, after what seems a slight sore
throat. On examining the fauces then, they are found
red and dry, the tonsils dripping with a thick, opaque,
offensive matter. Sometimes there is also great external
swelling of the throat.

Dr. Camps[1] believes that three distinct varieties of the
disease, if not three distinct diseases, have prevailed.
1. Cases which have presented a precise resemblance to
those described by Bretonneau. 2. Other cases present-
ing many of the characters of the Fothergill sore throat.

[1] Med. Times and Gazette, March, 1853.

3. Cases consisting in the sore throat accompanying scarlatina, whether the eruption has been present or not. The type of diphtheria, properly so called, is essentially asthenic.

Dr Pollock[1] conceives that Bretonneau had painted the disease too strongly. True diphtheria, so described, was not a prevalent disease, but many cases more or less approached it. All such arose from poisonous influences, and however different, were yet identical. In the same family these throat affections may approximate to and diverge from the diphtheritic type, there being in some exudations, in others ulceration and excoriation.

Mr. Bottomley,[2] of Croydon, remarks as follows:—

"It appears to me that at the commencement of the attack there is but a slight congestion of the mucous membrane of the pharynx, accompanied with slight constitutional disturbance; but in a few hours the membrane puts on a livid appearance, and runs rapidly into the gangrenous state; and that the false membrane is a deposit of layers of lymph in the early stage of the disease, which soon loses its vitality, and acts as an extraneous body, thereby preventing the parts from performing their natural functions, and, accompanying this change, great depression of the vital powers of the system takes place."

Mr. Thomas Smith, of Kent County, writes:—

"There are three forms in which the disease presents

[1] British Medical Journal, July, 1859.   [2] Ibid.

itself, viz: simple ash-colored diphtheritic membrane in patches, with very slight congestion of the surrounding parts, and without fetor; secondly, a deeper color, and more widely spread membranous exudation, with fetid breath, and intense engorgement of dark hue; thirdly, the membrane with much tonsillitis, in a few cases resulting in quinsy. But there has been a fourth and more formidable state of things to contend with, viz., an extension of the membrane, in either of the above forms, to the larynx and trachea. . . . Lately there has been more tonsillitis, and frequently superficial ulceration. There is a depression of the vital powers.

"In observing the progress of this epidemic, I have been instinctively led to reflect on the altered type of disease in general. I have myself no doubt of that alteration in the type of disease observed since the year 1832 in England."

Mr. Cammach,[1] of Bennington, remarks:—

"Diphtheria was epidemic in this district last year, in November and December, and has been so again since July. Diphtheria varies in extent from simple herpes of the lips or nose, which are covered with vesicles which burst, ulcerate, and heal in two or three days, to the most extensive inflammation and sloughing and ulceration of the cheek, the palate, and the pharynx; and more in children than in adults. It extends into the larynx and trachea, and kills by asphyxia. In the

---

[1] Lancet, Oct. 1858.

mildest form there is a tendency to ulceration beneath a white, loosely attached membrane. . . . In the worst cases its vesicular nature can be distinctly traced, for a few hours after its commencement, from the large patch within the cheek or upon the gum, which will slough like cancrum oris, to the more diffused bullæ upon the soft palate and pharynx."

Dr. Moncton, in a letter to the *Medical Times and Gazette*, June, 1857, says:—

"Diphtheria is a distinct disease, easily recognized, and not to be dreaded till such changes have occurred about the fauces and tonsils as it is impossible to overlook. A remote kinship there certainly is between it and scarlet fever, but identical they are not. . . . Though, as the diphtheritic membrane loosens and separates from the surface of the throat and tonsil, sloughing ulceration *may* ensue, I feel at present fully persuaded that diphtheria and cynanche maligna are not the same thing. . . The constitutional symptoms, at first altogether slight, become very real as the disease advances. The main feature is prostration, not typhoid at all—no coma, no sensorial disturbance throughout, no sordes, no heavy lurid look; and in many cases the practitioner, if not warned by previous experience, or a careful observation of the pulse, is surprised to learn that the patient he left with clear countenance, cheerful manner, and little suffering, a few hours ago, has just gone off, while casually sitting upright, in a fatal syncope. . . . The practical fact is, however, this, that after the fourth or fifth day a diphtheritic patient becomes the subject of very real asthenia, not so much perceived by the patient as discovered by the lax pupil and feeble pulse, and that this state is the one which, about the eighth day, is too apt to terminate in death."

Dr. Copeman, in an essay on diphtheria, recently published, remarks:—

"On turning our attention to the features presented by the present epidemic, we shall find that, as a general rule, the constitutional symptoms bear but little proportion to the local mischief, and the danger chiefly to be feared is the extension of the false membrane into tho larynx and trachea, so as to produce suffocation in the same way as in croup. . . .

"It is true that on the first appearance of the epidemic, in several instances it knocked down its victims at once, showing itself as a poison too powerful to give time for the development of any decided symptoms, either constitutional or local.' But this is a character common to almost all severe visitations of epidemic disease at their first onset, and, as I have said before, many of the patients who have since died from it have exhibited no very marked constitutional disturbance."

Thus it will be seen from these various accounts of the disease, as it manifested itself in Great Britian, that not only was a distinct loss of substance in the fauces frequently observed, but that the great prostration and general constitutional disturbance did not fail to attract the attention of almost every practitioner.

If the materials for a full and satisfactory account of the epidemics of sore throat which have prevailed in Great Britian are scanty, they are very much more so as regards our own country.

Dr. Douglas, of Boston, in the year 1736, published an account of the first appearance of a "sore throat distemper" in this country. This account is alluded to by Dr. Bard in his valuable paper.[1] The epidemic which he describes was very malignant, and was attended with erysipelatous appearances and highly putrid symptoms.

In the first volume of *Medical Observations and Inquiries*, published in London in 1771, is an extract from a letter from Mr. Cadwallader Colden to Dr. Fothergill, concerning the *throat* distemper, dated—Coldenham, New York, October 1, 1753. He says:—

"The first appearance of the throat distemper was at Kingston, an inland town of New England, about 1735. It spread from thence, and spread gradually westward, so that it did not reach Hudson's River till nearly two years afterwards. It continued on the east side of Hudson's River before it passed to the westward, and appeared first in those places to which the people of New England resorted for trade, and in the places through which they travelled. It continued to move westwardly, till, I believe, it has at last spread over all the British

---

[1] Researches on the Nature, Causes, and Treatment of Suffocative Angina, &c. By Samuel Bard, M. D., New York.

Colonies on the Continent. Children and young people were only subject to it, with a few exceptions of some above twenty or thirty, and a very few old people who died of it. The poorer sort of people were more liable to have the disease than those who lived well with all the conveniences of life, and it has been more fatal in the country than in great towns.

"In some families it passed like a plague through all their children; in others, only one or two were seized with it. Ever since it came into the part of the country where I live (now about fourteen years), it frequently breaks out in different families and places without any previous observable cause, but does not spread as it did at first. It seems as if some seeds, or leaven, or secret cause remains wherever it goes. When the distemper becomes obvious, it has the common symptoms attending a fever, except that a nausea or vomiting is seldom observed to accompany it.

"It is attended with a moist putrid heat, the skin being seldom parched. The pulse is usually low, but frequent and irregular. The countenance dejected, with lowness of spirits; no considerable thirst; the tongue much furred, and the furring sometimes extends all over the tonsils as far as the eye can reach. At other times, in the milder kind, the tonsils appear only swelled with white specks of about a quarter of an inch or half an inch in diameter, which are thrown off from time to time in tough, cream-colored sloughs. Sometimes all the parts near the gullet or throat are much swelled both inwardly and outwardly, so as to endanger suffocation, and frequently mortify; but most generally the swelling internally is not so much as to make swallowing difficult. Sometimes these swellings imposthumate. The last complaint is commonly of an oppression or strictness in the upper part of the chest, with difficulty of breathing, and a deep, hollow, hoarse cough, ending in a livid, strangled-like countenance, which is soon followed by death. This disease is not often attended with that loss of strength that is usual in other fevers; so that many have not been confined to their beds, but have walked about the room till within an hour or two of their death; and it has often appeared no way dangerous to the attendants, till the sick were in their last agony. Some died on the fourth or fifth day; others on the fourteenth or fifteenth day, or even later. When this disease first appeared, it was treated with the usual evacuations in a common angina, and few escaped. In many families, who had a great many children, all died; no plague was more destructive."

As we have before remarked, Dr. Samuel Bard, in 1771, gave a very faithful description of an epidemic of sore throat, which prevailed in New York. It will be seen in the extracts which we give from his treatise, that his opinions correspond with those of Bretonneau. He recognizes the analogy between this disease and croup, as well as the manner in which it spreads from the throat to the larynx. He observed it sometimes as simple angina; sometimes as angina complicated with laryngitis, and occasionally as laryngitis alone.

In general the disease was limited to children under ten years of age, though some few grown persons, particularly women, had symptoms very similar to it. Most of the persons attacked were observed to droop before they were confined. Usually, the first symptoms were a slightly inflamed eye, a livid countenance, and slight eruptions upon the face. At the same time, or very soon after, those who could speak complained of an uneasy sensation in the throat, but without much soreness or pain. Upon examination, the tonsils appeared swelled and highly inflamed, with a few white specks upon them, which, in some cases, increased so as to cover them all over with one general slough; this, however, although a frequent symptom, did not invariably attend the disease. The breath was not offensive, and deglutition but very little impeded.

These symptoms continued in some cases for five or six days without creating any alarm; in others, a difficulty of breathing came on within twenty-four hours, especially during sleep, and was often suddenly increased to such an extent as to threaten immediate suffocation. Generally, it came on later, increased more gradually, and was not constant.

This stage of the disease was attended with a very great and sudden prostration of strength, a very peculiar, hollow, dry cough, and a remarkable change in the tone of the voice. In some the voice was almost

7

entirely lost, and would continue very weak and low for several weeks after recovery. These symptoms continued for one, two, or three days, and greatly increased in those who died; purging in several cases came on, the difficulty of breathing became more marked, and the patient died apparently of suffocation. This commonly happened before the end of the fourth or fifth day. One child, however, lived under these circumstances to the eighth day. Shortly before he died, his breath and expectoration were somewhat offensive; "but this was the only instance in which I could discover anything like a disagreeable smell, either from the breath or expectoration."

In some cases, instead of the difficulty in respiration, very troublesome ulcers appeared behind the ears.

"These began with a few red pimples, which soon ran together, itched violently, and discharged a great deal of very sharp ichor, so as to erode the neighboring parts, and in a few days spread all over the back part of the ear, and down upon the neck."

In a few cases, swelling of the parotid and sublingual glands was noticed. Dr. Bard says:—

"I met with but two instances of anything like this complaint in adult persons. Both of these were women, and one of them had assisted in laying out two of the children that died of it. At first her symptoms resembled rather an inflammatory angina; but, about the third day, the tonsils appeared covered in some places with sloughs resembling those on the tonsils; her pulse was low and feeble; she had a moist skin, a dejection of spirits, and some degree of anxiety, though nothing like the difficult breathing of the children.

"The other was a soldier's wife, who, for some time before she perceived any complaint in her throat, labored under a low fever. Her tonsils were swelled and inflamed, and covered with sloughs resembling those of the children; but her breath was more offensive, and she had no suffocation.

"I have had an opportunity of examiuing the nature and seat of this disease from dissection, in three instances. One was a child of three years old. Her first complaint was an uneasiness in her throat. Upon examining it, the tonsils appeared swelled and inflamed, with large white sloughs upon them, the edges of which were remarkably more red than the other parts of the throat. She had no great soreness in her throat, and could swallow with little or no difficulty. She complained of a pain under left breast; her pulse was quick, soft, and fluttering. The heat of the body was not very great, and her skin was moist; her face was swelled; she had a considerable prostration of strength, with a very great difficulty of breathing; a very remarkable hollow cough, and a peculiar change in the tone of her voice. She was exceedingly restless; was sensible, and when asked a question, would give a pertinent answer; but, otherways, she appeared dull and comatose. All these symptoms continued, or rather

increased, until the third night, on which she had five
or six loose stools, and died early in the morning.

"Upon examining the body—which was done on the
afternoon of the day she died—I found the fauces, uvula,
tonsils, and root of the tongue interspersed with sloughs,
which still retained their whitish color. Upon removing them, the parts underneath appeared rather pale
than inflamed. I perceived no putrid smell from them,
nor was the corpse in the least offensive. The œsophagus appeared as in a sound state. The epiglottis
was a little inflamed on its external surface; and on the
inner side, together with the inside of the whole larynx,
was covered with the same tough white sloughs as the
glands of the fauces. The whole trachea, from the
larynx down to its division in the lungs, was lined with
an inspissated mucus, in form of a membrane, remarkably tough and firm; which, when it came to the first
subdivisions of the trachea, seemed to grow thin and
disappear. It was so tough as to require no inconsider-
able force to tear it, and came out whole from the
trachea, which it left with much ease; and resembled,
more than anything, both in thickness and appearance,
a sheath of thin chamois leather. The inner membrane
of the trachea was slightly inflamed; the lungs, too,
appeared inflamed, as in peripneumonic cases, particularly the right lobe, on which there were many large
livid spots, though neither rotten nor offensive; and the
left lobe had small black spots on it, resembling those
marks left under the skin by gunpowder. Upon cutting

into any of the larger spots which appeared on the right lobe, a bloody sanies issued from them without frothing."

Dr. Bard attributes the prevalence of the epidemic which he describes to a particular disposition of the air, or *miasmata sui generis*—

"Which more or less, according to particular circumstances, generate an acrimony in the humors and dispose them to putrefaction; and which have a singular tendency to attack the throat and trachea, affecting the mucous glands of these parts in such a way as to occasion them to secrete their natural mucus in greater quantities than is sufficient for the purposes of nature, and which in this particular species, when secreted, is really either of a tougher or more viscid consistence than natural, or is disposed to become so from rest and stagnation."

The disease he considered of an infectious nature. In the treatment bleeding was advocated, according to circumstances, and the use of mercury, gargles, fomentations, &c., as local remedies.

We have devoted much space to the remarks of Dr. Bard. But his little treatise has always been considered as very accurate and truthful in its delineations, and as a valuable contribution to medical science. His observations are quoted by almost all writers on this subject since his day, and particularly by Bretonneau.

Since the epidemic described by Dr. Bard, we do not find any other of a similar character mentioned by writers, until, in 1831, Dr. Bell speaks of having witnessed this affection in an epidemic form in Philadelphia. For the last few years, however, as in England, diphtheria has been much more frequently met with, and in some portions of the United States, especially in California, very fatal epidemics have prevailed. The medical journals in the various parts of the Union contain numerous descriptions of the disease as it has prevailed in certain sections. From a few of these we select extracts.

A terrible epidemic occurred at San Francisco, and in other towns of California, in the autumn of 1856. It had all the characters of pharyngeal diphtheria. Dr. J. V. Fougeaud[1] has published a monograph on this epidemic, in which he speaks of the mortality amongst children in several counties around the Bay of San Francisco as having "assumed an appalling character."

"Few children attacked by it recovered. The disease begins in a very insidious manner by a little engorgement or inflammation of the soft palate, pharynx, and one of the tonsils. (The attack seldom commences on both at the same time, but soon extends to both if not arrested.) At this period of the malady, the patient complains but little, there is often no fever, or it is very moderate. The pain in the throat is much slighter than in the usual forms of common sore throat, so slight in-

[1] Diphtheria: a Concise Historical and Critical Essay, &c. Sacramento, 1858.

deed, that the little patients go about playing as if nothing was the matter. In some exceptional cases, however, the fever and inflammation about the pharynx are considerable from the beginning. The character-istic signs of the affection soon follow this period of invasion. They consist in small portions (plaques) of white or yellowish lymph deposited on the soft palate, the tonsils, and the posterior part of the pharynx. The cervical and submaxillary gland becomes inflamed and swollen, and the pain in swallowing and opening the mouth is occasioned more by the engorged state of the glands than by the internal secretion of lymph. These deposits go on increasing in size more or less rapidly, and, in violent cases, in a few hours the whole cavity of the throat is covered by them. Generally one side is more affected than the other, and upon examination the glands corresponding with the parts affected will be found more swollen than those of the opposite side."

Dr. James Blake,[1] of Sacramento, in a memoir on this subject, says :—

"The first effect produced by the poison is evidently on the nervous system. Drowsiness, prostration, or oppression, are manifested by infants, or complained of by adults, and when the disease is prevailing, this desire of children to sleep at other than their usual hours should awaken our suspicions. The pulse is accelerated from the first, but generally soft and typhoid, although

[1] Pacific Med. and Surg. Journal, August, 1858.

in some cases it is for a few hours rather hard. The
temperature of the skin is raised, although it is seldom
harsh or dry, but frequently moist, or even covered
with profuse perspiration. There is seldom any pain,
rarely headache or backache. The tongue is usually
coated, edges red, and papillæ prominent. The appetite
may remain good, and the digestion unimpaired. If we
examine the throat, we may, even within twelve hours
after the occurrence of the first slight symptoms, find
the tonsil covered with a grayish, pultaceous exudation,
which rapidly extends upwards into the nostrils, and
downwards towards the larynx; and again we might
detect only a redness of the tonsil, and a small point of
exudation two or three days after the commencement of
the disease, and at a time when the symptoms of general
prostration had become alarming.

"Again, cases present themselves in which the
general symptoms and the anatomical lesions proceed
pari passu; but in almost every case that I have seen, I
have considered that death was the result rather of the
action of the poison on the system, than from obstruction
of the larynx. In from twelve to twenty-four hours
after the formation of exudation on the tonsil, we shall
generally find the cervical glands enlarged, and in pro-
tracted cases this enlargement may become so great as
to afford a serious obstacle to deglutition and respiration. I have seen cases in which I think death was
thus produced, when the patient might otherwise have
rallied from the effect of the poison.

"The duration of the disease is very uncertain. I have seen it terminate fatally in four days from the first ascertainable departure from perfect health, and this in a strong, healthy child, and I have witnessed it run along for two or three weeks, and then terminate fatally. The cases that arise from contagion, and remain exposed to the original source of contagion, I believe, as a general rule, run a more rapid course than the sporadic cases; thus we frequently find two or three children in the same family dying within a day or two of each other, although the sporadic case might have had the disease some days before the others took it. This is probably owing to the continued absorption of the poison in a state of concentration."

In a communication to the *Boston Medical and Surgical Journal*, Dr. L. N. Beardsley, of Milford, Conn., writes that—

"This disease [diphtheria] appeared in an epidemic form and with great mortality in this vicinity during the months of March and April last. It first made its appearance in Orange, an adjoining town (which is in an elevated situation, and is a remarkably healthy place, with a sparse population), and for a while was confined entirely to the scholars attending a select school in the village. . . .

"Fourteen cases out of fifteen, of those who were first attacked, proved fatal, in periods varying from six to twenty-four days.

"Most persons residing in the district where the dis-

ease first appeared sooner or later had some manifestation of the disease. The period of incubation varied
from five to twenty days. The lymphatic glands were
in many cases greatly enlarged.

"The first symptom of this disease—and it is one
which we have never seen referred to by any writer on
the subject—was *pain in the ear*. It was not only patho-
gnomonic, but prominent, and almost invariably present,
in every case that came under our observation, for a
day or two before the patient made the least complaint
in any other respect, and before the smallest point or
concretion of lymphatic exudation could be discovered
on the tonsils or elsewhere."

The tonsils were enlarged and inflamed, with small
points of lymphatic exudation upon them, which gradually spread upwards into the nasal fossæ, and downwards into the larynx and trachea. There was extreme
prostration, depression of the nervous system, feeble
pulse, &c., but in no case was there any mental disturbance. There was nothing peculiar in the treatment.

Dr. Beardsley's account is concise, and well drawn up.

In Albany, N. Y., diphtheria assumed an epidemic
character in 1858, proving very destructive. Dr.
Willard, of that city, in a paper read before the New
York State Medical Society, states that it first appeared
in April, 1858, although its greatest severity was in
the autumn. In a population of about 60,000 there
were 167 deaths. Of the whole number only three
were of adults, the remainder being of children, mostly

under twelve years of age. The deaths of females were
about one-third more than of males. One portion of
the city suffered more than another, but no satisfactory
connection was traced between the disease and any local
cause.

A few cases of diphtheria have also been observed in
Boston, Providence, New Bedford, Weymouth, and in
several other portions of New England, but there has
been no serious epidemic of the disease in this section of
the country, besides those we have mentioned.

There is reason to believe that the disease may
become more firmly established with us, as has been the
case in both France and England.

We have thus given some account of the epidemics
of "sore throat" which have prevailed in various portions of the world at different periods. On making a
comparison, it will be found that all these epidemics
possess certain characters in common, although pre-
senting occasional features of difference. If we study
them together, it will be also seen that they are closely
connected by a bond of union which is to be found in
the pathological anatomy of the disease, and which consists in a peculiar exudation. This was clearly recognized by Bretonneau, and is in fact the dominant idea
in his memoir upon the subject. Bretonneau was incorrect, however, as we have shown, in bringing together,
under the term diphtherite, affections which are separated by wide intervals; he was wrong in supposing
the absence of all constitutional symptoms in the disease

as also in regard to the integrity of the subjacent
mucous membrane on the removal of the exudation. At
least, we can truly say that his views on these points do
not coincide with what experience has taught us within
the last few years. So that, while we give M. Bretonneau the credit of having established these two leading
facts—viz., that all the various forms of epidemic sore
throat which have prevailed in different parts of the
world are identical, and that the characteristic of this
identity is the existence of the exudation—we must
confess that his description is wanting in many points
necessary to a faithful representation of the disease.

We subjoin portions of an article by MM. Barthez and
Rilliet, contained in their admirable *Traité des Maladies
des Enfans*, as also the brief definition by Dr. J. Copland
in his dictionary as being more comprehensive than the
description given by M. Bretonneau.

"The angina described by authors under the name of
gangrenous, pseudo-membranous, *couenneuse*, and to
which M. Bretonneau has applied the term diphtherite,
is a disease which principally attacks children, and the
character of which has given rise to numerous discus-
sions. It may occur as a primary disease (the true diphtherite of Bretonneau), and also as a secondary disease,
supervening most commonly upon eruptive fevers.

"*Pathological Anatomy.*—The uvula, tonsils, and pharynx are covered by false membranes of greater or less
thickness, of a yellow or yellowish-white color, and sometimes gray. They exhale no fetid smell after death, and

are generally very firmly adherent to the subjacent mucous membrane, especially in the pharynx and arch of the palate. The tonsils are rarely covered with a continuous layer, but spotted here and there with patches of various sizes, many of which penetrate into the lacunæ of these organs. In the pharynx, the false membrane forms a large plate, a sort of yellow covering to the mucous membrane, sometimes continuous, sometimes disposed in broken or interrupted layers. The false membranes have sometimes a gray color, which led for some time to the belief that they were the result of gangrene; but the gangrenous aspect of the pharynx is due to the putrid degeneration of the pellicular concretions themselves.

"The exudation of blood, which is not unusual in diphtheritic inflammation, completes the error. The false membrane, colored by this fluid, successively assumes different tints, marks of its decomposition.

"M. Bretonneau maintains that the mucous membrane subjacent to the exudation for the most part preserves its usual consistence and appearance. 'Slight ecchymosis, and a trifling amount of erosion upon the surface, in cases where the disease has been of long standing, constitute the chief alterations in the tissues.' In some cases which have come under our observation we have witnessed much more serious lesions; but, on the other hand, we have not met with those lines of ecchymosis which are described as being always present in the

8

pharynx and upon the velum palati. In two cases under our care the pharynx was deeply ulcerated.

"The tumefaction of the submaxillary glands is a lesion which M. Bretonneau considers as being almost constant. They attain a considerable size, but rarely suppurate.

"*Symptoms, &c.*—Diphtheria commonly sets in with slight febrile symptoms, the strength and appetite not being sensibly affected. The patient complains of a slight pain in the throat: no change in deglutition. Very shortly after the first attack, a slight swelling of the tonsils is observed, and frequently a little exudation of false membrane. Soon whitish or yellowish-white spots are seen on the tonsils, which extend to the larynx, velum palati, and pharynx. Sometimes these are limited to the tonsils and velum palati, when they often lose the white color, and become of a dirty gray, giving out an extremely fetid odor; an abundance of saliva is at the same time running from the corners of the mouth. The glands of the neck gradually become enlarged.

"At the end of a certain time, according as the membrane is more or less adherent, it commences to separate, and is thrown off. Or, remaining adherent to the mucous surface, it gradually grows thinner, and thus disappears.

"During the course of the disease, the appetite not unfrequently remains unimpaired. There is neither diarrhœa nor vomiting. If the disease terminates favorably, there remains only a slight redness about the throat. In the fatal cases, the inflammation extends from the fauces to the air-passages, thus giving rise to croup. Occasionally the disease assumes a typhoid character, a condition which has not been observed by M. Bretonneau. When diphtheria runs through its course without complications, it generally lasts from six to nine days; if croup intervenes, it may prove fatal in one or two days."

Dr. Copland, in his dictionary, defines diphtheria as follows:—

"Soreness, pain, and heat in the throat, often increased on deglutition; redness, with an exudation of a buff or gray-colored lymph in spots at an early stage, commencing either in the fauces, on the tonsils, or pharynx, and quickly extending to these, and often also to the larynx and œsophagus; the exudation becoming more continuous and firm, accompanied with fever, and appearing generally either epidemically or endemically."

If we carefully examine the various epidemics of diphtheria, we shall be able to bring them together under two principal forms of the disease—the mild and the severe.

The mild form is usually preceded by more or less fever, by some loss of appetite, a slight difficulty in deglutition, with, perhaps, some discomfort about the fauces. The tongue presents a thick whitish coat. On examination, at the very outset of the disease, the velum palati, uvula, and pharynx are of a bright red color. The tonsils are slightly swollen, and are of the same red hue. In a short time, generally from twelve to thirty-six hours after the attack, upon one tonsil, and sometimes upon both, are seen distinct white patches of exudation of false membrane. These soon extend over the uvula and posterior wall of the pharynx. The exudation adheres more or less firmly to the adjacent mucous surface, and cannot be easily removed. In a few cases the exudation remains confined to the tonsils, and neither grows black nor putrefies. The surrounding mucous membrane is swollen and projecting. The parotid and submaxillary glands are not much swollen.

The duration of the mild form of the disease is from six to nine or ten days.

In the severe form, the disease is ushered in by intense headache, hot pungent skin, rapid feeble pulse; there is great difficulty in deglutition, and the respiration is much hurried. The tongue is covered with a thick, dirty brownish coat. On examination of the throat, the tonsils are found enormously swollen and covered with a thick ash-colored membrane, which has also extended to the uvula and to the posterior walls of the pharynx, and not unfrequently gives out a fetid odor. Unless arrested by treatment, all the symptoms increase in severity, the respiration becomes much oppressed, there is a barking cough, and a change in the voice, which becomes hoarse and indistinct; the deglutition becomes so painful that children refuse to swallow even liquids; the saliva dribbles from the corners of the mouth, and an acrid discharge flows from the nares. The glands of the neck are greatly swollen and tender. The patient is restless to an extreme degree, tossing about and then sinking into a semi-comatose condition. These cases, when they prove fatal, as is the general rule, terminate either by rapid prostration of the vital powers or by an extension of the diphtheritic membrane into the air-passages.

M. Trousseau makes two divisions of the disease—simple and malignant diphtheria. In both, the essentials of the disease are the same. The one may generate the other, and the most simple case may give rise to another of the most malignant type.

Such, then, are the principal features of diphtheria. There are some points, however, as regards its nature, which require to be considered more in detail. First, the characteristics of the false membrane itself claim our special attention.

As regards the physical appearances of the false membrane, if closely examined by the unaided sight, it has the character of a fibro-plastic membrane. In the larynx it presents a whiter color than when it is situated in the fauces, and very much resembles the membrane thrown out in true croup, although it is softer and often soddened by the sanious matter which exudes from beneath and around it.

Dr. Jenner distinguishes two varieties of diphtheritic exudation, one of which is very tough and elastic, and as much as one-eighth of an inch in thickness, resembling washleather; the other, gray, pulpy, or creamy. The former consisting of such fibres as we see in the buffy coat of the blood coagula—the latter, pus pyoid corpuscles of Lebert and other smaller and larger granular corpuscles, epithelium and oleo-protein granules. Dr. J. teaches that these two forms of concretion are severally related, the latter with the asthenic, the former with the so-called inflammatory types of the general disease.[1]

After very long and careful examination, it has been observed that the exudation is preceded by a sero-mucous transparent liquid which in some cases is very abundant. This liquid once exuded, soon takes on more density and a closer adherence to the surface which secretes it, and at certain points becomes a little less transparent, assuming a yellowish tinge. These points soon run together, coalesce, and thus form a very thin pellicle, which may be regarded as the commencement of the false membrane. In fact, this commencement of the false membrane is an act of coagulation, according to M. Empis, which takes place by a precipitation of fibrin independently of any agency of the living tissue. This is to be seen most distinctly in the air-passages, particularly in the larynx and trachea, in which the tubular cast is seldom ever adherent, and is commonly much smaller than the cavity it occupies; its external surface, therefore, being separated by a considerable interval from the mucous membrane.

That coagulation is not determined by the mucous membrane is, in fact, shown by the experience of M.

---

[1] British and Foreign Med.-Chir. Review, 1862.

Empis[1] in cases where tracheotomy has been performed upon children. He says:—

"At the end of a few hours after the operation of tracheotomy, whatever care might be taken to clear the canula, the instrument was seen to be lined with a layer of whitish concretions, the thickness of which continually increased. These concretions were evidently only the result of the coagulation of the liquid by which the sides of the canula were constantly covered."

The pellicle thus formed, which we said may be considered as the first degree of the false membrane, is thicker at the centre than at the circumference, and generally may be easily lifted up, although in very small pieces, owing to its friability. Beneath this superficial pellicle, according to M. Empis, there is still an exudation of sero-mucous matter which gradually coalesces with the pellicle already formed, thus producing a false membrane several lines in thickness, and adhering very closely to the subjacent surface.

In many cases the membrane thus formed appears to remain for some time stationary, and then sooner or later it takes on an increase in thickness as well as in extent of surface. The secretion of sanious fluid which embues and softens the concretions is also augmented, becomes very dark colored, and exhales a fetid odor similar to that of gangrene. This especially applies to the deeper portions of the fauces, to the vulva, and to the anterior parts of the vagina.

[1] Arch. Gén. de Méd., Fevrier, 1850.

With regard to the cicatrization of the subjacent surface, and to the disappearance of the false membrane, M.
Empis[1] says:—

"We never see the membrane disappear all at once,
leaving in its place a cicatrized surface, as is the case
with an ordinary eschar, but it is by a gradual process
that the pellicle diminishes in thickness, in proportion as
the edges of the abraded surface cicatrize. If, however,
we modify the secreting surface by an energetic local·
treatment, we can cause the complete disappearance of
the membrane, leaving nothing beneath but a granulat-
ing surface of a healthy character."

The exudation is sometimes situated upon the cutaneous surface, at other times upon the mucous, and not
unfrequently upon both at once. Any portion of the
external surface of the body may become the seat of a
diphtheritic false membrane, the only condition essential being the absence of the epidermis, the skin thereby
approximating to the condition of a mucous membrane.
This cutaneous diphtheria has been much more
prevalent in certain epidemics than in others, especially
in France. In some the cutaneous affection has been so
frequent as to become the prominent characteristic of the
disease. Leech-bites, blistered surfaces, excoriations of
any part, various wounds, in the progress of an epidemic,
might become the seat of diphtheritic inflammation.
Whatever may be the situation of the exudation, it has
been incontestably proved that the diphtheritic affections

---

[1] Arch. Gén. de Méd., 1850.

of the skin are identical in their nature with those which are seated in the mucous membrane of the fauces and larynx. Nor is the external manifestation of the diphtheritic poison in any way less formidable than the faucial. In many cases reported by M. Trousseau, the symptoms of low typhoid were present; they often terminated fatally, or were followed by a long tedious convalescence.

When a wound is attacked by diphtheritic inflammation, it becomes painful, fetid, and discolored serosity pours from it in abundance, and a gray soft coating soon covers it with a layer of increasing thickness; the edges swell and become violet. The wound remains often obstinately stationary for months; sometimes it spreads; then an erysipelatous blush is seen around it; pustules form, become confluent, burst, and leave apparent a diphtheritic patch, which spreads even from the head to the loins.

A curious fact which has been observed as regards the seat of the diphtheritic exudation, is, that although it is found equally in the mouth, on the soft palate, the tonsils, the pharynx, the nasal fossæ, the larynx, trachea, and even in the bronchial tubes, on the conjunctiva, the vulva and anus, and upon the skin, it is not found upon those portions which are removed from the contact of the air; these seem refractory to the extension of the disease. M. Empis[1] remarks, that he never saw true diphtheria extend into the œsophagus, while, on the con-

[1] Arch. Gén. de Méd.

trary, the exudation of certain aphthous affections show a great tendency to spread into the œsophagus, but never into the respiratory organs. The atmosphere would thus certainly seem to exert an influence in promoting diphtheritic inflammation. The same observations have been made by M. Isambert,[1] as well as by others.

Mr. Smith directs the attention of the profession to an affection which in many respects resembles diphtheria, but which differs from it essentially both in its nature and its results. He gives the following as the characteristics of spurious diphtheria: The patient usually complains, first of a curious feeling in the throat, as if a pin were pricking it; there is languor with pains in the back and legs; and sometimes considerable tenderness on pressure on the outside of the throat, just under the angle of the jaw.

The tonsils and uvula are more or less tumefied, and of an angry red color, while on their surface there are small, irregularly shaped yellowish white spots. These, however, are evidently of an aphthous nature—there may be only one or two on the tonsil or on the uvula, or they may be very numerous. However great their number may be, their edges do not coalesce; each spot is isolated. They never look excavated, but seem as if they just floated on the mucus which moistens the throat.

The appearance of the tongue usually indicates

---

[1] Archiv. Gén. de Méd., 1857.

derangement of the digestive organs, and the pulse is smaller and more frequent than in health.

The treatment of spurious diphtheria is exceedingly simple; a mild aperient—10 or 15 drops of the tincture of the muriate of iron, three times a day, with a simple gargle of chlorine water, will be sufficient. The use of stimulants and a liberal diet will remove the prostration and muscular debility which may follow after an attack of this disease. Spurious diphtheria never proves fatal. Though accompanied with debility, it is not followed by paralysis or albuminuria; a patient who has suffered from this affection may afterwards have true diphtheria. The affection seems to be most common among young females.[1]

In order to determine the value of the exudation as a characteristic of diphtheria, it is well known that M. Bretonneau made numerous experiments relating to the effects produced by the application of irritant substances to the mucous membrane. As the result of these experiments, he found that no substance was capable of producing similar effects excepting cantharides. He says:—

"The action of the oil of cantharides when applied to the surface of the tongue and lips is almost instantaneous. In less than thirty minutes the epidermis shrivels and becomes raised and detached. It is soon replaced by a concrete pellicle, at first thin and semi-transparent, which speedily becomes more opaque and thicker. Like the

diphtheritic exudation, this membrane, which is at first
slightly adherent, is detached and reproduced with great
readiness. Within a period of six or seven days it may
be several times renewed."

M. Bretonneau concludes, from these experiments,
that the membrane of cantharides is anatomically identical with that of diphtheria, and is, therefore, forced to
admit that diseases cannot be distinguished merely by
their anatomical characters.[1]

"The facts relating to the cantharidic inflammation do
not in the slightest degree weaken the specificity of diphtheria; on the contrary, if we consider them in their
true light and in their complete development, they prove
it experimentally and demonstratively. However close
may be the resemblance between the two forms of inflammation, they are distinguished by well-marked characters. The cantharidic inflammation is limited to the
surfaces which have been subject to the inflaming action
of the vesicant, and soon become extinct; while it is in
the nature of the diphtheritic inflammation to extend
and to persist."

"With the view of determining how far the act of
fibrinous concretion may be considered a consequence
of the anatomical or physiological peculiarities of the
structure affected, independently of the constitutional
state, or of the morbid condition of the blood arising
from the disease, I made the following experiments: I

---

[1] Traité de la Diphthérite, p. 367.

injected into the air-passages of several dogs small quantities of a solution of cantharides in olive oil, and examined the consequent alterations of the mucous membrane after various periods. Two hours after the introduction of the solution, it was found that the mucous surface of the larynx was scattered over with patches scarcely perceptibly redder than the surrounding membrane, and that that structure was covered co-extensively with those patches, with a gelatinous covering of tolerably firm concretion, differing from that of diphtheria only in its greater transparency—a character, probably, mainly attributable to the absence of lamination—arising from its simultaneous formation. This concretion possesses a structure which is identical with that of the early condition of diphtheria, consisting of a fibrinous matrix or substratum, in some parts of which cells are imbedded. The substratum appears on microscopic examination to be transparent and faintly granular, but sometimes exhibits indistinctly the characters of fibrillation. . . . . The cell wall is of extreme delicacy, and incloses a spheroidal nucleus, distinguishable without the addition of acetic acid. (Fig. 2.) On the addition of that re-agent, the former becomes distended but does not disappear, while the latter either assumes the form of a spheroidal highly refractive body or is resolved into the double, triple, or horse-shoe shaped forms often described as characteristic of the pus-corpuscle. On examining the mucous membrane subjacent to the concretion, it was

9

found to have lost its columnar or ciliated epithelium, but the cells of the subjacent epithelial layer existed in an unaltered condition. They differed so completely in appearance, size, and structure, from the exudation cells,

Fig. 2.

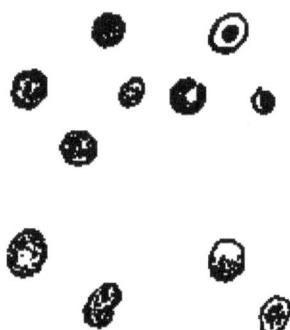

After Sanderson.

that there was no difficulty whatever in distinguishing them. In two days the process of transformation of the substance of the concretion into fibrous tissue had commenced. The pellicle possessed great firmness and elasticity, and could be stripped off the affected patches with ease to any extent.

"Of these facts, I will not further comment than to observe that the only important difference between the cantharidic and the diphtheritic concretion, consists in the absence of any tendency in the latter to transformation into permanent tissue, as contrasted with the early period, at which that process commences in the former. So far as concerns this mere fact of fibrinous concretion, we are perhaps entitled to infer that it indicates nothing more than the intensity of the process of exudation;

and that in diphtheria, the subsequent changes are prevented or retarded either by a morbid modification of the fibrin itself, or by an abnormal condition of the adjacent living structures." (Sanderson on Diphtheritic Sore Throat. *Brit. and For. Med.-Chir. Review,* Jan. 1800, pp. 181-9.)

Under the microscope the false membrane of diphtheria exhibits the ordinary elements of such structures, although its characters appear to vary somewhat. The elements usually detected are, chiefly, molecular particles, matted epithelium-cells of all kinds and shapes, pus, and blood-cells. These are arranged in layers, and united so as to form a membranous deposit.

Dr. J. Darrack states that he had examined a number of the patches of the membrane, which were carefully removed during life, and some after death. The elements found in all these examinations, were cells—young epithelial nuclear bodies, not affected by acetic acid, and most likely aborted epithelial cells, with pus corpuscles and granular matter—the granules occasionally assuming a disposition to form themselves into parallel lines. In no one case could be perceived a distinct fibrillation as is easily recognized in the transudations, upon the pericardium and other serous membranes. It is true that a granular form of fibrin has been described, but this has not been established.[1]

M. Empis has particularly investigated the pathological anatomy of the disease by the aid of the microscope.

[1] American Journal of Med. Sciences, 1861.

Now, it is well known that some observers, among whom
we may mention Vogel and Dr. Laycock, have associated
with the disease the presence of a parasitic fungus which
fixes itself on the mucous membrane of the fauces, and
is thought to be the starting-point of the vascular condition of which we have spoken, which afterwards gives
rise to the exudation. This parasitic fungus is the
oïdium albicans.

M. Empis, after noticing the statement of Vogel, that
the oïdium albicans is to be found in the pellicle of diphtheria, says:—

"This author has evidently confounded under the
term diphtherite all the pseudo-membranous exudations,
without examining into their nature or characters, for
this parasite is not found in the true diphtheritic or
fibrinous exudations, but only in those of muguet."

He then goes on to compare the diphtheritic exudation with other similar products, such as the buffy coat
of the blood, the false membrane of pleurisy, the exudation of blistered surfaces, and that which occurs in the
scarlatinal sore throat, and arrives at these conclusions:
That it is easy to determine, by means of the microscope—1st, the pseudo-membranous exudations of
muguet, which have nothing in common with other
false membranes; 2d, the buffy coat of the blood; 3d,
the false membrane of pleurisy; but that it is impossible
to draw any distinction, founded on microscopic investigation, between the exudation of diphtheria and that of

the blistered surface, or that which occurs in the angina of scarlatina.

As the development, then, of this parasitic growth takes place in a variety of other diseases, we must regard it as purely accidental, or at least secondary, and by no means as characteristic, or an exciting cause of the disease under consideration.

The communication of Dr. Laycock also fails to inspire us with that confidence in his theory which it would perhaps have done, had the case been one of uncomplicated diphtheria. Moreover, he himself also admits that this parasite is discoverable in the patches of aphthæ as well as in the secretions of the mouth in other diseases.

In an excellent communication to the *Medical Times and Gazette*,[1] Dr. Wilks says:—

"Opinions still vary as to the true nature of diphtheria, and therefore as to its connection with a parasite fungus (oïdium albicans). As on several occasions the white film on the throat has been found to consist of this fungus, it has been conjectured whether the malady is not one having a parasitic origin, and the belief has been rendered more probable from the fact that several new diseases have of late prevailed throughout the organic kingdom, both animal and vegetable, which are clearly traceable to parasites—for example, the oïdium of the vine. . . .

[1] October 2, 1858.

9*

"My attention being directed to this matter, I took the opportunity to examine the films which occasionally form on the mouths of those sick with various diseases; and on submitting them to the test of the microscope, felt some surprise in witnessing, in all, fungous growths, which I have not been able to distinguish from that of diphtheria."

After giving a brief history of several cases of different diseases, in all of which either a distinct pellicle or a thick secretion was present, Dr. Wilks says:—

"These facts are sufficient to show that a vegetable fungus may spring up on the buccal mucous membrane in various cases of disease, but requiring probably some previously morbid condition for a nidus. Is it not so in diphtherite? Is the disease, strictly speaking, a malignant sore throat, and the formation of a pellicle an accident, or is the latter an essential part of the affection?

"In speaking of the parasitic growth found in the above-mentioned instances, we are aware of the objection which can be made—that the fungus of diphtheria is peculiar (supposing it always to be present), and that found in the mouth of other sick persons is in connection with aphthæ, and is another variety. In answer, I can only say that I failed to discover in the above cases any difference, and, moreover, the character of the pellicle, and its rapid extension over the whole mouth, throat, and tongue, was totally unlike ordinary aphthæ."

Dr. Wade, of Birmingham, considers that there is present in some cases, in or near the exudation of diphtheria, a fungous growth—not, however, the oïdium albicans, but the leptothrix buccalis, such as is so commonly met with in the mouth and pharynx. Further investigations, however, have shown that the presence of either of these parasitical growths is to be considered as a mere accident, and not an essential part of the affection. In conclusion, we may say that the distinguishing character of the diphtheritic exudations, and that which separates them from other forms of exudation, is, "that they have the power of organization, and never become vascular. Hence they never concur in the reparation of tissue, but putrefy on the surface if they be not removed, existing always as a foreign body."

Is Diphtheria Infectious?—Upon this point, as we might naturally suppose, there is a wide difference of opinion. M. Bretonneau maintained that the exudation of diphtheria possessed a special virulence, and that the disease may be not only propagated by the application of the secretion from an affected surface to sound parts, after the manner of smallpox, but that, like syphilis, diphtheria cannot be communicated from a diseased to a healthy person in any other way. He says:—

"Innumerable facts have proved that those who attend patients cannot contract diphtheria unless the diphtheritic secretion in the liquid or pulverulent state is placed in contact with the mucous membrane, or with the skin on a point denuded of epidermis, and this application must be immediate.

"The 'Egyptian disease'[1] is not communicated by volatile invisible emanations, susceptible of being dissolved in the air, and of acting at a great distance from their point of origin. It no more possesses this quality than the syphilitic disease. If the liquid which issues from an Egyptian chancre, as visibly as that which proceeds from a venereal chancre, has seemed under certain circumstances to act like some volatile forms of virus, the mistake has arisen from its not having been studied with sufficient attention. The appearance has been taken for the reality."[2]

In support of his opinion, M. Bretonneau has collected a few cases. One is that of M. Herpin, who was surgeon to the hospital at Tours. A child attacked with diphtheria, who had also transmitted the affection to its nurse, was placed under his care. Upon visiting it one day, and during the process of sponging the pharynx, in a paroxysm of cough, a portion of the diphtheritic matter was ejected from the mouth, and lodged in the aperture of the nostril of M. Herpin. This he neglected to remove, and the consequence was a severe diphtheritic inflammation which spread over the whole nares and pharynx. The constitutional symptoms were extremely severe, and the prostration so great, that convalescence occupied more than six months.[3] Dr. Gendron, of Chateau de Loire, received on his lips portions of

[1] Considered by Bretonneau as identical with diphtheria.

[2] Traité de la Diphthérite.

[3] Arch. Générales de Méd., Jan. 1854.

diphtheritic exudation, expelled by a patient during a fit of coughing. Laryngeal inflammation came on with much violence, but his life was saved by prompt and decided measures.

In 1826, M. Bretonneau was summoned to the Ecole Militaire, in which diphtheria was prevailing; although many cases of the disease occurred, none proved fatal after his arrival. He states, however, that a boy affected with frost-bite of his foot, happening to use a bath that had been employed for a diphtheritic patient, became the subject of painful diphtheritic exudation on the great toe.

M. Lespieu[1] also gives an account of a soldier who, during the epidemic of the disease at Avignon, used the teaspoon of a diphtheritic patient, and in consequence contracted the disease in his mouth; and of another, who was attacked with diphtheria the night after sleeping with a patient.

Similar cases have been cited by authors in favor of the theory of contagion by inoculation. On the other hand, Prof. Trousseau failed in experiments which had in view the inoculation of himself and two of his pupils with diphtheritic matter, and Dr. Harley, of London, was not more successful in similar experiments on various animals.

M. Bretonneau goes so far as to maintain that the facts which he relates, and other details in his possession,

[1] Mémoires de Méd. et Chirurgie Militaire, Paris, 1854.

corroborate the assertion that the atmosphere cannot convey the contagion of diphtheria, which is only transmissible by inoculation. This opinion, however, is not supported by the experience of other writers, neither does it accord with the facts deduced from recent epidemics. In fact, it may be very clearly shown from the evidence already collected, that contagion plays the principal part in the propagation of diphtheria.

M. Isambert,[1] in his paper upon the epidemic of malignant sore throat, which occurred in Paris in 1855, gives the following as his experience:—

"Diphtheritic affections sometimes appear sporadically; they also often seem to be endemic, as well as epidemic and contagious. As predisposing causes, we may consider that the lymphatic temperament, a feeble constitution, privation, &c., all exert a decided influence. Youth is much more exposed to the disease than any subsequent age. Locality and overcrowding have a positive effect; so also do cold and changeable seasons.

"Epidemic influences are much the most powerful. As to the contagious nature of the disease there can be no doubt, since many physicians have contracted the disease. The opinion of M. Bretonneau that diphtheria is not transmitted by the atmosphere, but is always the result of inoculation, is altogether too exclusive. With M. Trousseau, we cannot reject infection at a distance as one of the means of propagation possessed by diphtheria."

[1] Archives Générales de Méd., 1850.

With regard to the influence exercised by the moisture of the air, by the temperature, and by the particular locality, M. Trousseau thus expresses himself:—

"In the villages of the Loire, remarkable for their salubrity and for their excellent position, I have seen diphtheria prevail to a terrible extent, while the villages of Sologne, situated in the midst of marshes, remained exempt; and, again, hamlets bordering upon ponds depopulated by the epidemic, while others enjoyed a complete immunity."

The observations of M. Empis lead him to favor the idea of contagion. While at the same time he recognizes, as a character of diphtheria, "the property which it has of being generalized in the economy, like the diseases *totius substantiæ*;" a property which, as he observes, may be best appreciated when the disease is studied epidemically.

Carnevale and M. Aurelius Severinus, as well as Franciscus Nola, admit the contagious properties of diphtheria, as well as almost all the writers upon the subject of the sevententh century.

Dr. Samuel Bard, as we have before remarked, considered the "suffocative angina" which he describes, as infectious.

"The disease I have described, appeared to me to be of an infectious nature, and as all infection must be owing to something received into the body, this, therefore, whatever it is, being drawn in by the breath of a healthy child, irritates the glands of the fauces and trachea as it passes by them, and brings about a change in their secretions. The infection, however, did not seem, in the present case, to depend so much on any generally prevailing disposition of the air as upon effluvia received from the breath of infected persons. This will account why the disorder should go through a whole family and not affect the next-door neighbor."

To come now to the observations of more recent writers upon this point, we may cite the remarks of Dr. Ranking in his admirable lectures on diphtheria,[1] to which we have already alluded:—

"My own conviction is, that it is infectious to a limited degree; by which I mean that when patients are accumulated in small, ill-ventilated rooms, the disease is likely to be communicated; but I do not fear that, like scarlatina or erysipelas, it may be propagated in spite of all sanitary precautions, still less that the infection can be conveyed by the clothes or persons of those who visit or superintend the patients. That it commonly spreads through the family once invaded is to be attributed, in some degree, to the persistence of the same cause as originated the first case. What that cause is, it is difficult to determine.

. . . . "Stench and poverty and crowded rooms have ever been the sad heritage of the agricultural laborer, but diphtherite is only of recent origin. Doubtless these insanitary adjuncts to a laborer's life predispose him and his children to the assaults of any epidemic malady, but the true and specific cause of diphtheria is a something superadded, and which our senses cannot appreciate."

In an article by Dr. Edward Ballard, of Islington (*Med. Times and Gaz.*, July 23, 1859), the following facts are given in support of the infectious character of diphtheria as it came under his own observation :—

"1. Infectious diseases habitually spread in families they invade. Out of 47 families there were only 15 in which the other members all remained healthy. Of course it may be argued, in opposition, that all the members of a family are equally exposed to the operation of local causes of disease.

"2. As a rule, it spread in the houses it invaded chiefly among those members of the several families who were most closely in communication.

"3. In no case where separation from the sick person has been effected early in the disease, have I noticed that it has spread to the separated individuals. In one case where communication had been allowed for three days before separation, a child was seized with diphtheria on the sixth day of removal from home.

"4. The following special instances (of which we give one) may be adduced of communication of the disease from one house to another :—

"Jane J., æt. 10 years, resided at Islington, with her mother, an aunt, and three sisters. On May 1st and 2d she was on a visit at the house of an uncle, whose daughter, Jane's cousin, was kept at home because she

10

was believed to have a cold. On the 2d, this child exhibited decided symptoms of diphtheria; the attack was
slight and she recovered.

"On May 6th, a servant in this house was taken ill
with a severe attack of diphtheria, and was removed to
St. Bartholomew's Hospital, where she died. On the 2d,
Jane returned home, was taken ill on the third with
diphtheria in a severe form, and died on May 9th. Her
mother and a sister, aged fourteen years, were both taken
ill on May 11th. She had not been so much with her
daughter as other members of the family up to the 8th,
when she sat up with her all night. The tonsil sloughed,
and there was a complete cast of the trachea expectora-
ted. She died on the 13th. The sister, who was also
attacked on the 11th, slept with her mother, and, when
not at school, was continually in and out of Jane's room,
sitting there sometimes for hours together. She died on
May 14th, asphyxiated. Another elder sister, who slept
with Jane and the aunt, suffered from nothing but a
slight sore throat."

The results of inquiries instituted at fifty-seven houses
where fatal cases occurred, with respect to local causes of
disease, were as follows:—

"In more than half the houses, then, which were examined there was some defect or other in the sanitary
arrangements or in the surrounding conditions of the
patients. In the greater number of the houses thus deficient, the fault was discovered in the state of the drain-
age."

Some writers of experience maintain that diphtheria possesses no contagious properties whatever, and others accord to it but comparatively feeble influence in this respect.

M. Daviot,[1] in a memoir on diphtheria, says:—

"Pharyngeal diphtheria is purely and simply an epidemic disease. Like other diseases which assume this character, it only manifests itself in those localities and individuals which have the most affinity for it. Springing from an alteration in the constituent elements of the atmosphere, an alteration unknown in its essence but appreciable in its effects, it is propagated through the medium of that fluid. . . . A great number of persons were struck by the epidemic a few days after arriving in the infected places, and without having communicated with any patient."

M. Daviot denies, as regards an epidemic which he describes, that it generally happened that all or the greater number of the members of a family were attacked at once, and states that it was quite as common that only a certain number of persons living under one roof were affected, while the successive attacks took place at considerable intervals. M. Daviot thinks such results can only be accounted for by—

"Similarity of organization and predisposition in individuals placed under the same hygienic circumstances, and, therefore, subject to the same morbific influences. . . . Will any one contend that the conta-

[1] Memoirs on Diphtheria (New Sydenham Soc.), London, 1857.

gious principle could have six months, a year, or even more of incubation before its development? Such an explanation is contrary to all probability, and does not require to be refuted."

M. Daviot did not meet with an instance where diphtheria was communicated by personal intercourse. He remarks that neither the attendants nor those who cauterized the throats of affected children contracted the disease. He concludes that pharyngeal diphtheria is not in itself contagious, and that it only appears to be so when associated with eruptive fever.

Dr. Crighton,[1] of Edinburgh, records the results of 45 cases of diphtheria occurring in his practice. Of these, 25 were males and 20 females; out of this number 9 proved fatal, or 1 in 5. Of these, 6 died of asphyxia with membranous exudation in the air-passages, and 3 by pure asthenia. They were instances of faucial diphtheria. In one case, aged 21 months, vulval diphtheria occurred. The mean age of the fatal cases was within a fraction of seven years.

" In only two cases was there anything like proof of contagion, and, from all that I have seen of diphtheria, I believe that, although it would be incorrect to separate it from the list of communicable diseases, yet it is very feebly so compared with many others. I may mention one instance which struck me particularly, where, in a large family of six or seven children, and chiefly under the age of twelve, a child had the disease in a very

[1] Notes on an Epidemic of Diphtheria. By R. W. Crighton.

severe form, and although he was never isolated during the day from the others, but lay on a sofa in a room where I generally found several of them at my visit, they all escaped."

Dr. Moncton (*Med. Times and Gaz.*, Feb. 26, 1857), after much experience in the disease during epidemics which prevailed in the county of Kent, says:—

"No decisive instance of its communicability has come before me; on the contrary, I have seen it attack individuals only, in a family of liable persons, much more frequently than I think scarlet fever would have done. My own conviction is, that diphtheria is epidemic, endemic (*i. e.*, largely affected by locality), and non-contagious, or, if contagious at all, vastly less so than scarlet fever, from which last it is very distinct."

Dr. Jenner, in his lectures upon the origin of diphtheria, draws the following conclusions:—

"First, that the disease is infectious; second, that the infected element does not require for its development any of the ordinarily considered antihygienic conditions; third, that the family constitution is one of the most important elements favoring the development of the disease and determining its progress; fourth, that it is very doubtful even if any of these hygienic conditions favor its development or give it a more untoward course when it occurs."[1]

---

[1] Diphtheria, its Symptoms and Treatment, by William Jenner, M. D. London, 1861, page 51.

Space would fail us, if we attempted to bring forward more than a very small portion of the argument and evidence which have been offered in favor of the contagious or non-contagious properties of diphtheria. There are, however, one or two points which we may consider further.

In connection with certian epidemics, especially in France, there were frequently observed cases of cutaneous diphtheria, which, from their persistence and superficial site, seemed peculiarly to favor transmission by contagion. As a general rule, this was never developed unless when the epidermis was raised or removed; and the observations of M. Trousseau, and others, have incontestably proved that the diphtheritic affections of the skin are of a nature identical with those which have their seat in the mucous membrane of the larynx and fauces.

Now, although those who favor the idea of contagion find in the phenomena of cutaneous diphtheria strong ground for the support of the theory of inoculation, there are facts which would seem equally to oppose it. For example, it has been observed in these epidemics, that the false membrane upon the skin not only presents itself in those not previously affected with faucial diphtheria, but it not unfrequently attacks remote parts, such as we should suppose were inaccessible to inoculation, as, for example, the folds of the groins in children, and the spaces between the toes. "A single well observed fact of this kind is sufficient to cast a doubt on the theory of inoculation."

Again, it sometimes happens, according to M. Trousseau, that diphtheria, especially when it occurs as a sequel to measles and scarlatina, is complicated with an eruption of bullæ of rupia simplex. These often become the seat of cutaneous exudation. As the bulla becomes flaccid from the absorption of its contents, instead of the formation of a thick brownish crust, it is observed that a firm concretion can be felt beneath the still entire epidermis.

The influence which meteorological and cosmic conditions exert in the production of diphtheria, is no better understood than is the relation existing between these same conditions and the production of other epidemic diseases.

Bretonneau, for example, had the idea that his diphtheria needed a damp atmosphere for its development. In the recent epidemics, both in France and in England, many instances are recorded where the disease prevailed in very dry and high situations. And in our own country, similar observations have been made. Dr. Wooster, in a monograph on diphtheria as it prevailed in California, explains how far the views of Bretonneau are applicable to the disease as it presented itself to his notice. He says:—

"In our climate the air in summer becomes so dry, that if an ordinary soft wooden pail or bucket, be half filled with water, and set in the sun in the open air for

six hours, and then two quarts of water be added, it will
leak through the joints of the shrunken staves, above the
surface of the first portion of water. A miner uses a
bucket to bail water from a hole all the forenoon, and,
although it is perfectly saturated with water, yet if he
leaves it in the sun while he goes to his dinner, when he
returns it will often fall to pieces as he attempts to take
it up.

"This is the kind of air in which the disease has
occurred with unequalled fatality in this State. In this
city I cannot ascertain that a case has occurred in that
part of the town built over, or near the waters of the bay,
or on the salt marshes near it. But I have seen cases in
the high part of the city, and on bluff headlands extending into the bay, points that, from their elevation and
constant exposure to a strong breeze, would be thought
inaccessible by any morbid effluvia."

In this connection, we cannot refrain from citing the
somewhat poetical, but at the same time very truthful
remarks of Mr. Ernest Hart.[1]

"It was observed of diphtheria in France, and it is
equally characteristic of its course in England, that it did
not obey any known climatic or meteorological laws.
It descended upon Tours, in the rear of the Legion of La
Vendée; it broke out in crowded and ill-ventilated barracks, and it spread throughout the town. It visited
alternately the open hamlets of the rural departments
and the crowded courts of the great cities. It raged in

[1] On Diphtheria, its History, &c., by Ernest Hart, London, 1859.

Orleans and in Paris, through the Sologne and in the Loiret. It reached the sea-side, and fell with violence upon the infant population of the city of Boulogne. It appeared to be equally independent of all atmospheric conditions. Was a theory formed that its intensity depended upon the solar influence, and that the heat of the summer months lent fresh force to its destructive attacks —soon it raged with greater violence in the winter months, and during the cold season. Was a connection traced between the localities of its invasions, and the marshy ill-drained character of the land—the next season it was found to ravage dry and elevated stations with equal rage. It has been no less careless of the limitations of heat, cold, dryness, and moisture, since it has established a camp in this country. * * * It has swept across the marshy lowlands of Essex, and the bleak moors of Yorkshire. It has traversed the flowery lanes of Devon, and the wild flats of Cromwell that are swept by the sea-breeze. It has seated itself on the banks of the Thames, scaled the romantic heights of North Wales, and has descended into the Cornish Mines. Commencing in the spring months, it has continued through the summer, and if extremes of temperature have appeared to lend it fresh vigor, and the heat of the dog-days, or the severe frosts and sleet of winter have fostered its strength, yet moderate temperature has not greatly abated its influence, and it has struck a blow here and there through all the seasons."

Without doubt, diphtheria, as well as other diseases of

a similar character, follow general laws, and in many cases we are obliged to confess our entire ignorance as to the exact nature of those laws.

But if we cannot ascertain the influences which govern these epidemics, perhaps on closer investigation we may discover certain individual or hygienic circumstances which may affect them either as direct or as predisposing causes. Thus, as a general rule, we shall find that diphtheria is more frequently associated with the ill-ventilated, contracted hovels of the poor, seizing by preference upon the unhappy subjects depressed by poverty and its attendant evils. Yet these are not the exclusive conditions for the development of diphtheria. We find in the various reports of these later epidemics that the disease has made its appearance, and carried off its victims, in the abodes of refinement and wealth.

"Zymotic in its nature, it tends to fasten upon whomsoever is debilitated by previous disease, or by a constitution naturally feeble and artificially effeminized, or whose vitality is lowered by the depressing influences of luxury, indolence, and inactivity; and the habitual defiance of physical and hygienic laws, which is so frequent an element in fashionable life. Hence individual causes come into play, and introduce this associate of the poor into the palaces and mansions of the great, which they so often fringe. Diphtheria finds there its victims pale and anæmic, or grossly sanguineous, and unhealthily excited."[1]

---

[1] On Diphtheria. By Ernest Hart, London, 1859.

Finally, all we can affirm is, that, as a general rule, anti-hygienic conditions of any kind favor the invasion of diphtheria, as well as of other similar epidemic diseases.

One element in the nature of diphtheria is of recent discovery. We refer to the presence of albuminous urine in the disease. The first observation upon the relation of albuminuria to diphtheria appears to have been made in connection with a case reported by Mr. Wade, of Birmingham, to the Queen's College Medico-Chirurgical Society in December, 1857, and afterwards published in his *Observations on Diphtheria.*[1] Shortly after this, during researches on this disease at Paris, MM. Bouchut and Empis made a similar discovery. Albuminuria did not exist in every case examined, but it was present in twelve out of fifteen cases. Both of these observers attach great importance to this renal complication, as affording an anatomical explanation of the cause of death, when this cannot be attributed to either of the other modes, viz., death by asphyxia or general poisoning. In fact, it was considered by them to indicate the infectious nature of the disease, in this respect resembling purulent infection, which is accompanied by a similar alteration of the urine. On this point M. Bouchut arrives at these conclusions. "Albuminuria in the absence of scarlatina or asphyxia (dependent on laryngeal obstruction) is a sign in diphtheritic diseases of a commencement of purulent infec-

---

[1] Observations on Diphtheria, by W. F. Wade, B. A. &c. &c., 1858.

tion, and coincides with a very great gravity of the disease." These conclusions he founds on the observations, that both in diphtheria and purulent infection there are, 1st, alteration of the color of the blood, which assumes a bistre tint; 2d, masses of pulmonary apoplexy, more or less numerous, similar to those which precede the development of metastatic abscesses; 3d, ecchymoses of purpura on the skin, or the serous membranes and the viscera. MM. Bouchut and Empis are of opinion that in addition to the preceding alterations, there is nothing farther necessary to establish the connection between these diseases but the presence of visceral abscesses, or purulent collections in the serous membranes.

In all the children under their care for diphtheria, the urine was analyzed both by heat and nitric acid. When albuminuria was present, the urine contained a very large proportion of salts, which rendered it cloudy and of a milky appearance at the moment of emission. At first, the heat caused the salts to be held in solution, when carried to a higher degree of heat, the albumen was precipitated. In three cases, the precipitate was very large, in the remainder, it was moderate in amount.

Together with albumen, Mr. Wade usually found in the urine tube casts and renal epithelium, the former being either "small waxy casts," or "epithelial casts." He is of opinion that albuminuria produces a diminution in the total amount of solid excreta, that is, that the special functions of the kidney are suspended, whereby symptoms arise which are indicative "of the retention within the system of those matters which should be excreted."

Our author has not informed us at what period of the disease he has first detected albuminuria, neither does he give any observations tending to show how far the progress of the disease is affected by the condition of the kidneys, which would seem to be indicated by the presence of "casts," &c., in the urine.

More recently, Mr. Wade, in speaking of this subject, remarked that the changes are more commonly microscopical, consisting of crowding and opacity of the epithelium, which is most readily detached and rapidly disintegrates. Casts of various kinds are to be found in some specimens of the albuminous urine of diphtheria. Apart from its early occurrence, there seems to be a special tendency to albuminuria, about the seventh or eighth day, at which time the disorder has a natural tendency to terminate. Under such circumstances it is to be looked upon as a critical phenomenon. It may occur at any period.

Diphtheritic albuminuria is often preceded by urine of high specific gravity. The supervention of albuminuria may fail to reduce this. Mr. Wade therefore recommends the ingestion of bland fluids in as great quantity as the patient will take—half a pint every hour or two, if possible, in the case of adults.[1]

In a paper, communicated to the *British and Foreign*

<hr>

[1] Lancet, Aug. 23, 1862.

Med.-Chirurgical Review, Jan. 1860, Mr. Sanderson, upon the basis of eight cases, is not inclined to admit either of the doctrines advanced by Mr. Wade. He says:—

"In eight cases in which I have had the opportunity of making repeated observations as to the condition of the urine, the only ones which occurred to me since my attention has been directed to the subject, it has been albuminous in all."

Dr. Sanderson, having given a brief report of each of these cases, goes on to remark:—

"Although in several of the cases above related the cessation of albuminuria was clearly coincident with the amelioration of the patient, and the disappearance of the most alarming symptoms, it is not less certain that in one or two others albumen existed in large quantities in the urine, although the cases maintained a mild character throughout. From this it may be inferred that albuminuria is not in itself so alarming a symptom as M. Bouchut is inclined to imagine."

As it appeared of importance to Dr. Sanderson to ascertain whether the existence of albuminuria coincided with the solid excreta of the urine, he directed his experiments to that end. He offers, however, only one satisfactory observation, the following:—

CASE VI. W. D., male, aged 80. Albuminuria first observed about the eighth day; disappeared three days after; abundant.

General character of symptoms.—Extremely grave;

excessive prostration; intense adynamia, with nervous agitation and busy delirium. Concretion not examined. *Result—recovery.*—Slow convalescence, with extreme muscular weakness.

During a period of about nine days the albuminuria continued. During this time observations were made as to this condition of the urine. Without giving the two tables of analysis, we come directly to the result.

"At the acme of the disease, when the urine was intensely albuminous, when there was complete anorexia, and the ingesta were reduced to a minimum, the quantity of urea excreted in a period of twenty-four hours was about twice as great as that excreted during a similar period when convalescence was established, and he was eating with an appetite the ordinary diet of the hospital, with extras.

"The above facts show that diphtheria agrees with the other pyrexiæ in being attended with a marked increase in the excretion of urea, and that the existence in the kidney of the condition which is implied by albumen and fibrinous casts in the urine, does not necessarily interfere with that increase in the elimination of nitrogenous material. There is, therefore, no reason to apprehend the occurrence of uræmia as a consequence of the renal complication in diphtheria; this complication not being the cause of the dyscrasia, but merely the index of its existence."

With reference to the presence of albuminuria in diphtheria, there have been but few accurate observations made, and, in fact, until comparatively recently, it was thought that one distinctive mark of diphtheria, over other kindred diseases, was, that there were no albumen and no dropsy present. Certain it is that albuminuria has manifested itself throughout almost the entire course of grave cases of diphtheria, and which have yet terminated favorably. On the other hand, cases have occurred which have proved fatal when it has been absent.

There can be no doubt of the serious character of this renal complication, but further research and observation are necessary before we can ascribe to it any settled prognostic value.

In this connection we may also speak of the remarkable after symptoms of diphtheria, which have been observed by almost every practitioner who has had even a limited experience during the epidemics of the last few years, and which have been particularly referred to by MM. Trousseau and Bretonneau, and also by M. Faure.

After apparent recovery from the immediate effects of the disease, in many cases there still seems to be lurking in the system a morbid poison, whose special affinity is for the nervous system. Thus, prominent among the sequelæ of diphtheria, is paralysis in its various forms, more frequently local than general, also otalgia, amaurosis, headache, ophthalmia, &c. Epidemics of this last have been observed in Germany, and were described by Graefe in 1854,[1] and, in France, by M. Jobert in 1857.[2]

[1] Gazette Hebdomadaire, 1856.   [2] Archives Générales, 1857.

The most frequent form of paralysis has been that of the soft palate. The symptoms are a nasal twang in the speech, incapacity for suction, and the regurgitation of fluids by the nostrils. This form was thought both by M. Trousseau and others to be local in its origin. * But further observation has led them to change their views.

M. Trousseau makes the following clinical remarks:—

"The pathology of the paralytic affection was, for a long time, altogether misunderstood both by himself and others. In consequence of its being more frequently local than general, in other words, the palate and pharynx being more usually affected with paralysis than the system generally, he was for a long time under the impression that the loss of power was dependent upon the inflammation of the coats of the nerves supplying these parts, and on infiltration producing pressure on their motor muscles. A more extensive experience, however, of the general character of the paralysis which accompanies and follows diphtheritic affections, caused him to change his views, and he now believes that loss of power and sensibility is the direct consequence of the peculiar diphtheritic poison acting generally on the system, and strangely modifying the blood. He further stated a fact which has often come under his observation, that many children who have been subjected to the operation of tracheotomy fall victims to paralysis of the epiglottis and larynx."[1]

¹ Med. Times and Gazette, Jan. 27, 1859.

Again, in a communication to the *Gazette des Hôpitaux*, 1860, M. Trousseau remarks that this affection may be analogous to what is observed in certain cachexias. One curious circumstance in diphtheritic paralysis is the temporary extinction of venereal desire, which occurs at a very early period, even in those possessed of considerable genital ardor.

In a paper read before the Royal Med. and Chir. Society, March 24, 1863, Dr. Greenhow remarked that he had observed nervous affections were more frequent after the worst cases of diphtheria, and to bear some proportion even to the local severity of the attack; he had noticed that the paralysis and anæsthesia were sometimes more complete on that side of the fauces which had been most severely affected by the primary disease; he had found that a brief period of convalescence had almost always intervened between the disappearance of the sore throat and the accession of the nerve symptoms. This seemed important, as it went far to show that paralysis could not be entirely attributable either to the albuminuria, which often accompanied the acute stage, or to the anæmia, which closely follows it, as patients had often got rid of the former symptoms, and had begun to get strength and flesh before the accession of paralytic symptoms. These nerve affections are progressive in the same set of muscles, but do not attain their maximum of intensity even in the same set of muscles. The muscles of the fauces are the earliest and the most frequently attacked, and sometimes the only ones; next, impairment of vision, probably due to paralysis of the ciliary muscles, appeared to be the most frequent of the nervous disorders consequent on diphtheria: a great majority of sufferers from these nerve affections recover. As to treatment, Dr. Greenhow advised generous diet, rest in bed, &c. He considered nux vomica and strychnine as very valuable remedies after the complete development of the paralytic symptoms.

In the *Med. Times and Gazette*, January 4th, 1860, M. Royer makes the following statement :—

During the year 1860, there were 200 cases of diphtheria at the Hôpital des Enfans, in Paris; paralytic symptoms followed in thirty-one of these cases. The proportion was really greater, several children having been removed from the hospital prior to the period at which consecutive symptoms are usually developed. M. Royer believes that these cases of secondary paralysis are as rare in the other acute diseases of children, as they are common in diphtheria. Of forty cases of diphtheritic paralysis, which have come under his notice, the most frequent age was from four to six years, there being 21 female to 17 male infants. In almost all cases, the paralysis has commenced by the pharynx and velum palati, as shown by the nasal twang and dysphagia. Its occurrence would seem to be a proof of a greater amount of blood poisoning. The usual appearance is from the fourth to the eighth day; its mean duration is about a month. As a general rule, the prognosis is not unfavorable. Tonics, iron, sulphurous preparations, and the application of electricity constitute the chief treatment.

A paper was read before the Prussian Association for Scientific Medicine, in May, 1861, by Dr. Ebert, upon the subject of diphtheritic paralysis, which gave rise to an interesting discussion. Dr. Ebert referred to cases recently published by Bouillon La Grange, in which not only the soft palate, but also vision, smell, taste, and touch, the throat, œsophagus and the limbs had been paralyzed; and then related a case which had fallen under his own observation. Dr. E, believed that such palsies originated in the same way as rheumatic paralysis, and that a cold would be sufficient to produce paralysis in a patient who had suffered from diphtheria. Prof. A. Von Graefe denied that there was any connection between common paralysis and the diphtheritic disease; cases of paralysis occurred after every grave disease of the nervous system, as typhoid fever, erysipelas, &c. It was not difficult to trace the origin of the paralysis in diphtheria, as the nervous system was greatly affected. Every disease which was accompanied by fever, was also accompanied by paralysis of accommodation, and a semi-paralytic state of most of the muscles of the eye. If the large number of epidemics which had been observed in France was considered, the number of cases of paralysis was very small when compared with the frequent occurrence of palsy after other grave diseases.[1]

M. Maingault finds that the impairment of vision

---

[1] Med. Times and Gazette, May, 1861.

comes next in order of frequency after the affection of the soft palate. It varies in duration from a few days to six months, and in degree from the mere inability to read small print to perfect blindness. The ophthalmoscope yields no information; its sudden accession and rapid disappearance lead us to regard it as purely neurotic.[1]

Dr. Wade remarks (*Lancet*, Aug. 23, 1862) that paralysis, may follow as a kidney complication, and may attend slight, as well as severe cases of diphtheria.

In one case under his observation the paralysis has lasted two years, and may be considered as permanent.

Dr. Jenner, in his work on diphtheria, observes that the heart is the organ next in order of frequency to manifest disordered innervation; the patient dies from a literal asphyxia. In some cases, the paralysis is more widely extended: in these recovery is rare, death ensuing as from general paralysis.

But it is to Dr. Faure that we are more particularly indebted for the most complete account of these remote consequences of diphtheria. He describes this peculiar condition of the system

"As a state characterized by a gradually increasing loss of power, showing itself especially in all those functions connected with muscular movement. In some instances, several sets of organs are affected, in others only one, while again in others, the whole system is involved in the general debility. But whatever are the

[1] Brit. and For. Med.-Chir. Review, 1862.

variations in this respect, there is no definite relation
between the severity of the primary symptoms of diphtheria and that of the sequelæ. The primary symptoms,
though very formidable, do yet by no means of necessity
prove fatal; while, on the other hand, the comparative
mildness of the attack will not justify an absolutely
favorable prognosis, since death sometimes follows where
everything had seemed to warrant the most confident
expectation of recovery."

Several cases are given by M. Faure, in illustration of
the various phases of this condition, and he sums up as
follows:—

"Some time after an attack of diphtheria, from which
the patient has so completely recovered that no trace of
false membrane is left behind, the skin grows more and
more colorless without apparent cause, so that at length
it assumes almost a livid pallor. Severe pains begin at
the same time to be felt in the joints, the patient loses
power over his limbs, and soon sinks into a state of
indescribable weakness. At the same time, the disorders
that appear in different functions show that the various
organs which should minister to them are involved so
far as they are dependent upon muscular power. In this
respect, however, the phenomena are not constant, for
sometimes it is one set of organs, and sometimes another
which suffers most from this weakness. Very generally,
in consequence of the want of muscular power, the
patient becomes unable to sit upright, or does so with
great difficulty, while the legs cannot bear the weight of

the body; all the movements grow uncertain, tottering, hesitating and apparently purposeless. Very remarkable disorders show themselves also within the throat, for the velum is completely paralyzed, and hangs down like a flaccid lifeless curtain, which interferes with speech and deglutition. All the muscles of the jaw, neck, and chest are partially paralyzed in consequence of which mastication is rendered difficult, and the food can be neither easily moved about in the mouth nor readily swallowed. Vision is impaired, squinting is not unusual. The sensibility of the skin is much diminished, in the limbs it is sometimes completely lost, though morbid sensations, such, for instance, as formication, are sometimes experienced. Œdema of the various parts often occurs, and occasionally parts, here and there, lose their vitality, and become gangrenous. No general reaction occurs; fever is rare. The features grow duller and more and more expressionless, though a foolish smile sometimes crosses them, or now and then a ray of intelligence appears. Some patients have frequent fainting fits. As the condition goes on from bad to worse, the weakness becomes extreme, and death at length follows some fainting fit, or takes place when exhaustion has reached its uttermost; life, as it were, quietly, almost imperceptibly, passing away."

Such are some of the most common sequelæ of diphtheria. It is not to be understood, that in these cases a fatal termination is necessary, nor that the symptoms are necessarily so severe as have been depicted by Dr. Faure.

Further observations will undoubtedly clear away much that is obscure upon these singular after-effects of the disease. Even in our present state of knowledge of them, they certainly furnish materials towards the solution of the question—the identity or non-identity of diphtheria and scarlatina.

These cases are to be treated on tonic principles. The nervine tonics are especially indicated. In cases of local paralysis, astringents, feeble cauterization, and electricity may be employed.

Recent observations have shown, that clots in the heart may undoubtedly occasion the sudden deaths which are sometimes witnessed in diphtheria. Dr. Thompson calls the attention of the profession to this fact, in a communication to the *London Med. Times and Gazette*, Jan. 1860, and in the *American Journal of the Med. Sciences* for April, 1864, Dr. J. F. Meigs, of Philadelphia, reports three cases of death from this cause.

Our knowledge of the nature of diphtheria may be summed up in the following words:—

Diphtheria is a *specific* disease. This fact is shown by its origin, its progress, its manner of termination, and its sequelae.

Its diagnostic sign is the formation of an aplastic membranous exudation upon any portion of the cutaneous or mucous surface which is exposed to the contact of the atmosphere.

It is propagated by infection and contagion, and is both epidemic and sporadic in its invasion.

Its characters plainly indicate that it belongs to the category of *blood diseases*.

It is not allied either to cynanche trachealis, or to scarlatina.

The treatment is to be directed to the control of the exudation, and to the support of the constitution by means of tonics, stimulants, and by a nutritious diet. Of this we shall speak next.

Treatment.—Like all diseases which have prevailed epidemically, and which have appalled by their severity and fatality, or perplexed by their novelty, diphtheria has been subjected to a great variety of treatment. It is only within the last few years that anything like unanimity has existed in the profession in regard to this important point. Not to go back further than the period of Bretonneau's memoir on this subject, we shall find that an activity of treatment prevailed which would scarcely coincide with the ideas of the present day. Bleeding, both local and general, blisters, certain local applications to the pharynx, rapid mercurialization, formed the treatment in all cases. Mercury, in fact, was considered as the sheet anchor by a great majority of medical men. To quote the words of Dr. Bard: "But although I consider mercury as the basis of the cure, especially in the beginning of this disease, I do not by any means intend to condemn or omit the use of proper alexipharmics and antiseptics." Although a few practi-

12

tioners may still make use of this therapeutic agent, it is now generally agreed that such is the asthenic nature of the disease at the present day, that depletion is not borne well in any form, neither is the action of mercury defensible either in theory or practice.

As we are still unacquainted with any specific capable of arresting the course of diphtheria, our treatment must be directed simply to the conducting our patient in his progress through the disease. In the first place strict attention to certain hygienic rules is necessary. The most scrupulous cleanliness of person and surroundings, free and uninterrupted ventilation should be insisted on. If there are children in the family where the disease breaks out, the well ones should be sent away, or at least should be kept out of the room where the infected individual lies.

Mr. Wade recommends that the patient in all cases should be clothed in a flannel gown and kept in bed. I believe that the adoption of this plan would have saved almost innumerable lives.[1]

In the very early stages of the disease, if there is much heat and engorgement about the throat, cold wet compresses may for a time give relief. As the disease progresses, warm fomentations, and emollient applications generally, may be substituted. Blisters are to be avoided, both on account of their adding, by their irritation, to the engorgement and to the cellular infiltration, and

[1] Lancet, Aug. 23, 1852.

on account of their liability to take on a diphtheritic or sloughy appearance. As everything in the aspect of the disease, from the first, indicates that the powers of life must not be lowered, but on the contrary that the tendency to prostration must be averted in every way, neither leeches nor local bleeding are admissible, except perhaps in very rare exceptional cases. In certain epidemics, there is also danger that the punctures might take on a sloughy character.

Many practitioners commence the treatment of diphtheria with the administration of an emetic or a purgative. Under certain circumstances an emetic may be advisable, particularly when there is an early tendency to croupal symptoms. For the purpose, full doses of ipecac are preferable. Anything like purging, however, is to be sedulously avoided on account of the asthenic nature of the disease. The bowels may be moved by simple enemata, or by some mild laxative.

There are occasional cases of diphtheria so mild in character that local applications to the fauces may be sufficient, but as a general rule it is conceded that the disease requires a tonic and sustaining treatment, particularly is this the case at a late period of the disorder. In cases at all severe, the tendency is to depression and to death by asthenia, unless earlier terminated by asphyxia.

Stimulants and nourishment should be commenced with early, and persisted in systematically. The amount, of course, must depend upon circumstances, but in order to insure efficiency, they should be varied, and given in small doses at regular and frequent intervals; if rejected by the stomach, they should be given in the form of enemata. So also with respect to children, when they are frightened and distressed by painful attempts at swallowing, and absolutely refuse everything, we have the same resource.

Injections of beef-tea, with brandy and quinine, may be employed, and thus life be not unfrequently sustained, when otherwise it would inevitably have been extinguished.

With regard to the particular form of internal tonics, there is a variety of opinion. There are some which, perhaps, promise a greater chance of success than others, among which we may mention quinine, tinct. ferri chloridi, and chlorate of potash. But as each of these has powerful advocates in its favor, we imagine that, provided the strength of the patient be sustained, it is of little importance by which of these tonics it is accomplished.

The tincture of chloride of iron seems now to be preferred by the great majority of practitioners, on account of its unquestionable usefulness in the more asthenic forms of disease. The dose is from 10 to 15 drops, in water, every three or four hours.

"Of the many internal remedies which have been advised, we do not know of any on which so much reliance can be placed as on the tincture of sesquichloride of iron, with chlorate of potass, chloric ether and hydrochloric acid in the form of mixture, sweetened with syrup, full doses being employed according to the age of the patient, and frequently repeated. A free use should be made of generous wine, beef-tea, coffee, eggs, in combination with brandy and wine, milk, and whatever other form of nutriment the ingenuity of the surgeon or the fancy of the patient can suggest."[1]

Quinine may be administered in mixture, with or without the dilute hydrochloric acid, or in the form of pill; the dose and frequency of repetition must be governed by circumstances. If the chlorate of potash be preferred, it should be given in doses of from four to eight grains, according to age, in a bitter infusion with two to five drops of the dilute hydrochloric acid.

We come now to speak of the auxiliary measures to be adopted in the treatment of this disease, and first, of the local applications to the fauces. The propriety of these has been called in question by some writers, on the ground that the disease is a constitutional one, and, therefore, that they can be of no service. But there can be no more reason why the local remedies are not as applicable to this affection as in other constitutional diseases, for example, as in syphilis, scrofula, carbuncle, &c. In an excellent paper by Dr. Bristowe,[2] on the treatment of diphtheria, the following reasons are given for discarding heroic applications to the fauces:—

[1] Lancet, Sanitary Commission.
[2] Med. Times and Gazette, Sept. 1859.

"1. That the throat affection is merely a local evidence of a constitutional disease, which is unlikely to be arrested in its progress by any treatment directed to the secondary manifestations only. 2. That the throat affection rarely kills, except by involving organs, such as the trachea and deeper tissues of the neck, which are beyond the region of the possible influence of such agents. 3. That if the theoretical correctness even of such treatment be admitted, the application of remedies to the surface of a thick false membrane, with the hope that they may affect the subjacent mucous tissue, is not only clumsy, but, as regards the object intended, practically useless; and that the prior forcible removal of the membrane from the entire surface, in order to their efficient employment, is unjustifiable in the early stage, even if possible, and is likely only to be followed by increased inflammation, and reproduction of false membrane. . . . Of course, if a gangrenous state of the tonsils, or any other local complication, supervenes, such topical applications as are commonly had recourse to in like conditions of the throat should be employed."

While we concur in the remarks of Dr. Bristowe so far as regards the forcible removal of the false membrane, particularly in the early stages, the experience of almost all medical men of the present day bears witness to the efficacy of the application of caustics or escharotics to the throat.

M. Trousseau remarks that topical medication is, *par*

excellence, the treatment, notwithstanding the opposition to it.[1]

Mr. Wade maintains that interference with the false membrane will not prevent its reproduction, nor will it prevent laryngeal complication. We are justified in interfering with the throat exudation when there is excessive fetor, or when it is so copious as to interfere with respirations or deglutition, not otherwise.[2]

"Local treatment," says Dr. Greenhow, "applied to the throat internally, has been almost universally adopted in the treatment of diphtheria; and though I by no means deny its value when judiciously employed, I am sure much mischief has been produced by its indiscriminate use, especially by the tearing away of the exudation by probing or similar contrivances for the application of nitrate of silver or of strong caustic solutions. Observing that removal of the exudation, and the application of remedies to the adjacent surface, neither shortened the duration nor sensibly modified the progress of the complaint, but that the false membrane rarely failed to be renewed in a few hours, I very soon discontinued this rough local medication to the tender and already enfeebled mucous membrane. The propriety of this course became evident at the very first post-mortem examination I had the opportunity of witnessing, and has been confirmed by all my subsequent experience. In the first place, the application can but rarely extend to the entire diseased surface, and, in the next, the subjacent

tissues are so deeply involved in cases of really malignant diphtheria, that any application to the surface of
the mucous membrane could apparently exercise no
beneficial influence upon the disease. . . . . The
only instance in which much benefit can be expected
to arise from the local application of escharotics, is
when the patient is seen at a very early stage of the
illness while the throat is simply inflamed or the exudation, if it be already present, is circumscribed fully in
view and surrounded by healthy tissue."[1]

On the other hand, some writers maintain that the
disease at the outset is a local one, which rapidly brings
on a general *intoxication*. This would be a still stronger
argument—if we granted this to be true—for these very
local remedies, if applied in season, might prevent a
further extension of the disease.

There are a multitude of substances which have been
employed as local applications to the fauces, each of
which has its special advocates. During the last four
years the nitrate of silver, either solid or in solution, has
been perhaps more extensively used than any other substance. This, when used early in the disease, seems in
many cases to check the progress of the exudation; yet
it does not answer the purpose altogether, and further
experience has somewhat diminished confidence in it.
Indeed, in some instances it is a question whether the
free application of this caustic does not rather add to the
evil.

---

[1] On Diphtheria, by Dr. E. Headlam Greenhow.

"I have mentioned that I thought that the indiscriminate mopping of the fauces, as it is called, with solutions of nitrate of silver, was frequently attended with injurious results in this disease, principally, I believe, for this reason, that, owing to the struggles of the little patient, it is impossible to apply the caustic solution with that precision which the case absolutely requires. Thus, it is applied to parts which are entirely free from disease. I have been told of cases where the inside of the cheeks has been covered with it; in coughing, a portion of it has been expelled upwards through the nose, corroding the susceptible surface of its mucous membrane; and, again, other portions of it have seemed to pass downwards into the pharynx and œsophagus; and I am not sure that, during the convulsive struggling of the patient in resistance, some of it may not also enter the larynx, where it may possibly initiate those inflammatory changes in the mucous membrane of the air-passages which are too frequently the harbinger of death in this disease."[1]

Still, if carefully and properly used, nitrate of silver, in many cases, is undoubtedly of benefit. If in solution, it is to be applied by means of a probang or brush, swabbing over the diseased surface quickly, at the same time thoroughly. The strength of the solution should be from 30 to 60 grains, and perhaps higher, to the ounce of water, according to circumstances. For chil-

[1] Observations, &c., by F. A. Bulley, F. R. C. S., Med. Times and Gaz., April, 1859.

dren, a full-sized camel's-hair brush is best. The child should be placed on the lap of an attendant, and the head firmly fixed. If he will not open the mouth, the nostrils should be closed for a few moments, and as he opens the mouth for breath, the jaw should be at once depressed, and then, the tongue being kept down by the finger, the fauces are brought well into view, and the solution thus thoroughly applied. The utmost gentleness and patience should be exercised; but at the same time, it should be done with firmness, for upon the effectual accomplishment of this proceeding the success of the treatment will greatly depend. This should be repeated every three or four hours, so long as it is necessary.

The nitrate of silver may also be employed in the solid form, but this we should not advise, particularly in the case of children. During the struggles of the little patient the crayon might become broken, an accident which has happened, and fragments fall into the œsophagus or larynx, giving rise to serious lesions. Moreover, the nitrate of silver in this form has the disadvantage of creating a more decided eschar than the solution, simulating the diphtheritic exudation, and thus hindering the perception of the progress of the disease.

The tinct. ferri chloridi is an excellent substitute for the nitrate of silver, and is now generally preferred by a great majority of practitioners both in this country and in Europe. This may be applied by means of a brush or sponge, or in a gargle of the strength of two drachms to eight ounces of water.

The hydrochloric acid may be useful in some cases, and has also been extensively advocated. It is to be applied in a similar manner to the other substances of which we have spoken. In the case of children, the addition of honey to the acid is desirable. This is a favorite topical remedy of M. Bretonneau. He says:—[1] "At the commencement of the epidemic at Tours, topical remedies suggested themselves. The beneficial effects of hydrochloric acid soon gained for it an exclusive preference. In the use of this acid, it is preferable to employ it in full strength, at long intervals, than to return to less energetic applications more frequently."

Another gargle, which is very efficacious, and which has also the advantage of correcting the fetor of the breath and the secretions of the throat, is a solution of the chloride of soda, in the proportion of one drachm to six ounces. This may either be employed by itself, or combined with other applications. The same may be said of the chlorate of potash. The combination of chlorate of potash and hydrochloric acid with the tincture of the sesquichloride of iron is strongly to be recommended, especially in the croupal cases, the chlorate of potash having an undoubtedly anti-diphtheritic influence, where time permits it to be brought into play.

Numerous other applications to the fauces have been advocated and successfully employed. Among these

---

[1] Traité de la Diphthérite.

may be mentioned, strong solutions of sulphate of copper; the chloride of sodium, either by itself or combined with vinegar; gargles of tannin, capsicum, &c.; Monsell's salt in powder. Of this last substance, Dr. Beardsley, in his paper upon the epidemic at Milford, Connecticut, to which we have previously referred, writes:—

"Monsell's salt was found to be the most efficacious and valuable of all topical remedies, affording in some instances decided relief. Its active astringent property rendered it peculiarly appropriate, and well adapted to obviate that relaxed and enfeebled condition of the throat which attends the advanced stage of the disease."

In cases where there is much tonsillitis, we may employ the inhalation of steam, mucilaginous gargles, warm fomentations, &c. These often afford marked relief, and are useful adjuncts to the other treatment.

M. Grand Boulogne states that, in the Havannah, during two violent epidemics, he met with great success in the use of ice as a remedy. He caused the patients to keep it constantly in their mouths even into convalescence.

M. Bouchut[1] advises the ablation of the tonsils early in the disease, not only for the purpose of removing the exudation which appears on them, and which he considers the localization of the disease, but also of facilitating respiration. Such a proceeding we should not consider advisable, to say the least, for the following rea-

---

[1] Gazette des Hôpitaux, 1858.

sons: In the first place, the exudation is almost sure to re-form upon the cut surface; next, there is a great risk of severe hemorrhage; and finally, any cutting operation, however simple, had better be avoided, if possible, especially upon young children, and in a disease so asthenic in its character.

The removal of the tonsils in this disease might possibly be practised upon an adult, when there is great tumefaction, and for the purpose of facilitating respiration, and for this purpose only.

When the nasal fossæ have become implicated, various solutions should be injected through the nostrils. MM. Bretonneau and Trousseau recommend a solution of alum, or the insufflation of the same substance in powder. We should advise, however, a solution of the chloride of soda, in the strength of two drachms to eight ounces of water, to which two ounces of glycerine may be added. Frequent injections of warm water and soap may also be thrown up, in order to cleanse the parts and remove the offensive odor.

Nitrate of silver, sulphate of zinc, and, in fact, any solution which is applicable for the fauces, will answer a good purpose for injecting the nasal fossæ.

But when in spite of all means of treatment, energetically and judiciously employed, the disease progresses steadily onwards, and the larynx and trachea are invaded by the exudation, giving rise to symptoms of imminent danger, then the important question of tracheotomy must be entertained.

13

Without going into a history of tracheotomy, or a recapitulation of the arguments on the one side or the other, we most unhesitatingly say that, under the circumstances above mentioned, this operation is a resource which we are in duty bound to afford our patient, and in view of what experience teaches us is otherwise certain death. It is not that, by so doing, we increase his chances for life solely, but in the case of an unfavorable termination, we render his last moments less distressing.

It has been urged that the operation of tracheotomy is not warrantable in those cases of croup which are the result of the extension of the diphtheritic exudation to the larynx, as the patient not merely dies from asphyxia, but sinks likewise from a constitutional infection; on the other hand, it has been urged that there is even a better chance of success with the operation than in true croup, the membrane being less apt to spread to the bronchi.

For ourselves, we can see no validity in any arguments which have been adduced either in favor of or against tracheotomy in diphtheria, which would not be equally applicable to the same operation in cases of croup, and in this opinion we are supported by statistics.

With a view to a correct appreciation of the subject, we would refer to the remarks made by Dr. Fuller, in the course of a paper read to the Royal Med.-Chirurgical Society, in 1857. Dr. Fuller began by referring to the difference existing physiologically and pathologically between idiopathic inflammatory croup, and the diphtheritic form of the disease which commonly prevails in

France, and he pointed out that the objection usually urged against French statistics of tracheotomy in croup, viz., that diphtheritic cases are much more favorable for the performance of the operation than the croup cases usually met with in Great Britain, has no foundation in fact. By reference to 483 cases in which tracheotomy had been performed for the relief of croup in France, he showed that the operation had been eminently successful in the hands of French surgeons, and he reminded the society that inasmuch as the condition of the throat externally and the nature of the accompanying fever in diphtheritis are by no means favorable to the operation, the success which has attended it can be explained away only on the supposition often put forward by English writers, that in France the disease seldom extends into the trachea and bronchi, and is rarely accompanied by bronchitis or pneumonia. The fallacy of this supposition was, however, shown by reference to the recorded results of the post-mortem investigations of 311 cases of croup in France, and he also showed that in regard to its pathological effects, diphtheritis, when accompanied by croupal symptoms, does not, as compared with inflammatory croup, present any greater prospect of success for the operation than it does in the character of its accompanying fever, or the condition of the throat externally.

Granting then that the two diseases, inflammatory croup and diphtheria, stand on an equal footing as regards the applicability of the operation, let us briefly consider a few of the objections which have been brought against tracheotomy.

It is urged that the small amount of success which has hitherto attended the actual performance of this operation in croup renders it an expedient to which it is scarcely justifiable to have recourse. If we refer to the statistical inquiries of different countries, we shall find that this objection has no foundation. Thus, in France, where in cases of croup tracheotomy has been resorted to on an extended scale, although the rate of mortality has, on the whole, averaged about seventy-six per cent. of the cases operated upon, yet in about 680 cases in which the operation was performed, the mortality only amounted to sixty-eight per cent.

According to M. André, during the year 1856, there were 54 operations of tracheotomy for croup at the Children's Hospital in Paris. Out of these there were 39 deaths and 15 recoveries, or over 27 per cent.

The proportion of recoveries obtained by M. Guersant in a very considerable number of operations performed during the last three or four years was about one-third.

In a summary drawn up by M. Bouchut, he says :—

"Although the success of tracheotomy is not very striking, yet the results are such as ought to encourage its adoption. Thus M. Bretonneau performed the operation in 20 cases, and out of these 6 were successful. In my own practice, 160 operated upon, 5 saved. M. Velpeau saved 2 in 10. M. Petit, 6 operated upon, of which 8 were successful. Thus, out of 176 cases, we have 18 which terminated favorably."

M. Chaillou, in the *Journal of Practical Medicine and Surgery*, gives the following statistics as regards the operation in cases of confirmed croup. In eight years, 380 operations of tracheotomy were performed, of which 86 were successful, an encouraging result, when by far the greatest number of patients were operated upon in the last stages.

The statistics of tracheotomy at the Hôpital des Enfans in 1855 showed ten cures and thirty-eight deaths, out of forty-eight cases, or one patient saved in five. Since this period the ratio has very much improved, owing to a more extended experience in the mode of performing the operation, and in the necessary after-treatment.

In Great Britain the recorded results of the operation exhibit a fair amount of success. In 22 recorded cases in 1857, no less than eight terminated satisfactorily.

Dr. Fuller, above cited, reports five cases of croup for which tracheotomy was performed, in two of which life was saved. The results of the operation in England are, however, for some undetermined cause, far less favorable than those which have been obtained in France or in this country.

The most recent statement of the results of tracheotomy in France, is that of MM. Roger and See;[1] this

---

[1] Gazette Hebdom., Nov. 1658.

gives 126 recoveries in 446 operations; or 27 per cent. during the last seven years.

A much larger amount of statistics might be added to those which we have brought forward, but sufficient has been offered to prove the propriety under certain circumstances, of performing tracheotomy in this disease.

It has been objected that the operation was a very difficult one, and that in itself it was very dangerous. In answer to the first of these objections, we will say that, in the case of young children, it is often a difficult proceeding, and requires a greater amount of operative skill and care than is commonly supposed. These circumstances, however, should scarcely be held to militate against our having recourse to the operation when the necessity of the case demands it.

But that tracheotomy is in itself a very dangerous operation, the tendency of the evidence on this point goes to disprove. Thus, M. Trousseau[1] has collected the records of ninety-six cases, in which tracheotomy was performed for the removal of foreign bodies in the wind-pipe, and in seventy-three of these a complete cure was effected, the rate of mortality after the operation amounting to about twenty-four per cent. of the cases operated upon. This gentleman has himself performed tracheotomy in more than 200 cases, with success in more than a quarter of the whole number of cases.[2]

Dr. Gross, in his *Treatise on Foreign Bodies in the Air-*

[1] "Discussion at French Academy," by M. Trousseau.

[2] Brit. Med. Journal, Jan. 1862.

Passages, has collected the particulars of 176 cases in which foreign bodies had accidentally gained entrance into the air-passages. In 68 of these, tracheotomy was performed, and the mortality reached only 11 per cent.

We must take into consideration, when making a comparison between the results of tracheotomy performed for the removal of foreign bodies, and those of this operation for the relief of croup, that, in the former case, the tissues operated upon are generally healthy, whereas, in the latter case, they are the seat of certain morbid changes. Yet notwithstanding this, there is not sufficient danger in the operation itself, under any circumstances, to deter us from performing it.

Dr. West, after speaking of the more favorable results of the operation obtained in France than in England, owing, as he thinks, to its frequent performance in the former country when other means might have been tried which would probably have controlled the disease, says:—

"Still, if these facts detract something from the apparent value of the operation, they at least show that in itself it is not attended by serious danger; and recent statistics prove that, in as far at least as the diphtheritic form of croup is concerned, there is no sort of connection between an increased frequency in the performance of tracheotomy and a higher mortality from the disease."[1]

The gravest objection which is brought against the operation, is, that it is apt to induce severe bronchitis, or

[1] Lectures on Diseases of Childhood, &c., 1859.

at least to greatly aggravate any previously existing inflammation of the lungs or bronchial tubes. In answer, we say, that, although there is some ground for this accusation, on the other hand, it must be remembered that these very inflammatory conditions are the almost invariable complications of croup, however treated, and that they do not ordinarily follow tracheotomy when resorted to in other circumstances, as for the removal of foreign bodies, for acute laryngitis, or for œdema of the glottis.

Other objections have been brought against the propriety of tracheotomy in cases of croup and diphtheria, which we could satisfactorily answer did space permit. We can only add, in conclusion, that there do not appear to be any evils attendant upon the operation which counterpoise the indisputable benefits to be derived from it.

A few words upon the proper period for performing the operation. Tracheotomy has been, and is still considered by a great portion of the profession, especially in this country and in Great Britain, as the very last resort. Within the last few years, however, the opinion of those best able to form a judgment has materially changed. A middle period should be selected for the operation. We should not wait until the case is desperate, the patient in a complete state of prostration, in fact moribund; nor, on the other hand, should we attempt the operation too early, before other remedies have been fairly and completely tested. But we are to resort to the operation "so soon as ever we feel that our remedies are too tardy to overtake the disease."

There are some circumstances relating to the proper management of the operation and to the after-treatment, which greatly influence the results of tracheotomy, at which we must hastily glance. The first of these concerns the size of the tracheal tube, the importance of which was first insisted upon by M. Trousseau. This gentleman explains the occasional sudden and apparently causeless disappearance of the amendment which at first follows the operation, by the inadequate size of the canula, which is frequently employed, and which does not provide for the constant and permanent admission of a sufficient quantity of air. In illustration of this fact, M. Trousseau says:—

"Take a quill, and, closing your nostrils, endeavor to breathe entirely through it; at first you breathe easily enough, but soon your respiration becomes laborious, and at length you are fain to throw away the quill, and with open mouth once more to fill your lungs completely. Now precisely this is what happens when an opening of inadequate size is made into the trachea, air enters readily, and without the interruption which the spasm of the glottis occasioned; but it does not enter in sufficient quantity, and hence the return of the symptoms and the patient's death."

Acting on this principle, M. Trousseau makes a larger opening into the trachea, and introduces a larger canula than was formerly used; and this practice is now gaining ground, especially in the United States.

Dr. Hillier says, in a clinical lecture on Diphtheria, that in order to give the child an opportunity of coughing and clearing the tubes of mucus and other matters, the tube may be closed for two or three seconds by the finger. When the finger is removed a deep inspiration is taken, then the tube is closed again until an effort to cough is made, then the finger is suddenly taken away and the offending materials are expelled. Use a good sized *double* tracheal tube.'

Another necessary precaution has reference to the necessity of insuring to the patient, after the operation, a warm moist atmosphere, which may be easily effected by filling the room with steam from some simple apparatus; and to keeping the room at a fixed temperature, and, though well ventilated, free from all draughts. The neck also should be surrounded with several folds of muslin, so as to cover the orifice of the tube. Great care should also be taken to keep the canula free, and as upon this one thing the whole result of the operation may depend, it should not be intrusted to unskilful hands, but to a medical student, or to some competent person, upon whom full reliance can be placed. This is a point which has not attracted the attention which it deserves, for not unfrequently cases occur where death suddenly takes place from the stoppage of the tube, the persons in charge fearing to do what the occasion of the moment demands.

' Med. Times and Gazette, April, 1862.

Medical treatment must not be suspended after the operation. The same measures which were considered useful before the operation must be steadily persevered in. Great stress has been laid by a few writers in our country upon the importance of throwing nitrate of silver injections into the trachea. These we certainly advocate, as cases have come under our observation where very beneficial results have followed their employment.

The period at which the canula ought to be removed is also an important point, on account of the irritation of the edges of the wound which its long continued presence is apt to produce. M. Andró, in his statistics before alluded to, has endeavored to ascertain the proper period for this purpose. His observations were made in 17 cases. In 1 it was taken out on the fourth day; in 5 on the sixth day; in 2 on the seventh; in 3 on the eighth; in 1 on the eleventh; 1 on the thirteenth; 1 on the fourteenth, and 1 after the fourteenth. From the fourth to the fifth day is the time recommended by M. Andró. After the removal of the canula the wound is to be covered with a bit of gauze, the edges touched daily with the nitrate of silver, and dressed with a little spermaceti or other ointment. The tube is to be replaced if dyspnœa recur.

In addition to what has been already said on the treatment of diphtheria, it may not be inappropriate to give a summary of the treatment recommended by some of the principal practitioners of Europe.

Mr. Ranking, in his lectures on diphtheria (*Lancet*,

January, 1859), recommends the tinct. ferri chloridi, 10
to 15 drops every three or four hours, and the same to
be applied locally; the diet to be nourishing.

Mr. Hart, of the "*Lancet* Sanitary Committee," advises
a tonic treatment, tinct. ferri chloridi, chlorate of potash,
&c.; and as local treatment, the nitrate of silver, 30 to 60
grs. to the ounce, or the muriatic acid.

Dr. Kingsford (*Lancet*, Nov. 1858), in simple diphtheria, uses a calomel purge in the commencement. Then
chlorate of potash, with dilute hydrochloric acid in a
decoction of bark, and mopping the throat two or three
times a day with the compound solution of alum. In the
severe forms he uses wine and nutritious diet freely, and
gives tinct. ferri chloridi, with chlorate of potash, 10 to
30 drops of the former with 10 to 30 grs. of the latter,
every two or three hours, according to circumstances.
Nitrate of silver to the throat—wine and nutritious diet
freely. If much difficulty of deglutition, enemata of
strong beef-tea, and port-wine every two hours, the
quantity to be injected not to exceed two or three ounces
at a time. Mercury he thinks contraindicated, except as
a cachectic at the beginning.

Dr. Perry, of Kent (*Med. Times and Gaz.*, March, 1859),
gives oil of turpentine, ten drops every second hour, to a
child of from two to six years of age, and alternates this
with five grains of carbonate of ammonia every two
hours. Besides this, port-wine, porter, and beef-tea, or
wine with the yelk of an egg, *ad libitum*. He thinks
that mercury hastens the fatal result.

Dr. Cammack (*Lancet*, Oct. 1858) gives a calomel purgative where symptoms of laryngitis appear, and a decoction of cinchona with hydrochloric acid. A gargle of salt and vinegar for the mouth and throat, which he also injects up the nostrils when they become affected. He applies the solid nitrate of silver to the exudation. He is convinced that the malady is herpetic.

The editor of the *Lancet* (October, 1858) thinks the disease is not a new one, but believes it to be a form of scarlet fever. He gives ammonia and beef-tea early, and keeps the skin softened by the steamed blanket. A warm blanket wrung from hot water is to be put around the patient, this to be enveloped in dry blankets, and the patient to be sweated for an hour and rubbed rapidly dry, and again covered with dry blankets. "Keep him up with ammonia and good nutritious broths."

Mr. Thompson (*Brit. Med. Journal*, June, 1858) advises thorough applications of nitrate of silver to the throat, a stimulating gargle of nitrate of potash, and capsicum, or solution of chlorinated soda. Mild but continued counter-irritation over the upper part of the chest appeared of great service. General treatment he thinks of little use. Stimulants are often required in the early stage.

M. Roche (*L'Union Médicale*, July 26, 1859) places great reliance on the following treatment. Having first freely cauterized the false membrane with lunar caustic, he injects every hour against the fauces a solution of common salt, not of sufficient strength to create nausea.

14

The tincture of iodine he also employs as a topical application.

Mr. Ramskill (*Lancet*, February, 1859) makes use of an infusion of chamomile to wash and syringe out the throat and nares of children, to which he adds a few drops of creasote, or of the liquor calcis chlorinatæ. Internally he gives chamomile with muriatic acid and ether and quinine, at the same time good nourishment and stimulants.

Dr. West, in his *Treatise on Diseases of Childhood*, adopts the following mode of treatment. A drachm of the nitrate of silver to the ounce of water is applied to the throat either by means of brush or probang; if necessary, afterwards the strong hydrochloric acid, diluted with from four to ten parts of honey. One, or at the most, two applications of the stronger caustics in the twenty-four hours suffice. These are preferable to the weaker ones, as these latter must be applied frequently, which distresses the child. For this reason he does not make use of the tincture of iron, nor does he employ insufflations of powdered alum or calomel. The mouth may be kept free from the secretions which are apt to accumulate in it by syringing it every three or four hours, with a lotion of the chloride of soda, half an ounce to six ounces of water. As constitutional treatment, he advises quinine with the tincture of bark and hydrochloric acid, at short intervals. The best of nourishment and stimulants.

Dr. Semple (*Lancet*, October, 1858) says that the best

treatment is the application of strong caustics, of which the concentrated hydrochloric is the best, at the very earliest possible period. Nourishing diet, &c.

M. Empis (*Arch. Gén. de Médecine*) advocates the use of local remedies, such as the hydrochloric acid and the nitrate of silver, and for constitutional treatment, tonics and nutritious food. In these views M. Isambert also concurs.

In our own country, during the epidemic which prevailed at Albany in 1858, gargles containing chlorates of potash and soda, or vinegar with the mineral acids and tonics internally, constituted the principal treatment. During the epidemics at San Francisco, very much the same treatment was pursued. So also in Connecticut.

Prof. Chapman, of New York, in a series of excellent papers upon this disease, advocates the adoption of a stimulating treatment. He gives the history of thirty-eight cases in which the disease is presented in almost every varied phase. He says: "Of the remedies that have been employed in diphtheria, two only have proved themselves in our hands worthy of confidence, with the exception, in the chronic stage, in favor of the salts of iron. These two remedies—alcohol or cinchona in one of its forms—are administered in such doses and at such intervals as to secure one effect—the fullest stimulation of the nervous and vascular systems. Either singly may suffice when the vital force needs but slight aid to maintain the integrity of the blood; but the two united have more than a double power, and call out the greatest possible amount of resistance, since the nerve centres and bloodvessels, the great life-factors, are exalted to the highest point; although liquors, when given in such quantities and intervals as to occasion and keep up a steady, but not excessive excitation, not only quicken the functional offices of each organ, but act more especially on the nervous and vascular systems.

...... "It is a noteworthy fact that, in my experience, the diphtheria never attacks those habituated to the use of spirits. This, if confirmed, may be more than a remarkable coincidence. ..... Both the cinchona and the alcoholic stimulant, whether used singly or united, should be given with regularity and in sufficient doses to obtain their full effects; and then the latter, in a lessened quantity, continued for two or more weeks after the disappearance of the disease and its sequelæ. From the outset to a permanent restoration to health, one or perhaps both of these remedies are to be continuously administered."[1]

Although there is some diversity in the treatment of diphtheria, as laid down by different authorities, still, it will be seen that the affection is considered by all as one decidedly adynamic in its character, and that consequently a supporting treatment is necessary, and all depletory measures are to be strictly avoided. Authorities are also united upon the necessity of a more or less

[1] Practical Observations on and the Treatment of Diphtheria. By E. N. Chapman. Boston Med. and Surg. Journal, Feb. 1863.

energetic local treatment, particularly in the early stages of the disease.

Before closing our remarks upon the treatment of diphtheria, we must say a few words upon *tubing of the glottis.*

The unquestionable efficacy of tracheotomy under certain circumstances suggested the idea of inserting into the larynx through the mouth an instrument which might replace the canula of tracheotomy and render unnecessary the use of the knife. Although others had tried the experiment, M. Bouchut was the first who put it to practical use.

The operation consists in inserting into the larynx a metallic tube, which is to be retained for a longer or shorter time according to circumstances.

The instruments used are: 1. Curved male catheters of different sizes, open at both ends, and intended to penetrate into the larynx (*C, C*). 2. Straight cylindrical silver rings (*A*) of from ½ to ¾ of an inch long. provided at their extremities with two ridges at the distance of a quarter of an inch and pierced with a hole for the passage of a silk thread (*B*), the function of which is to preserve a hold upon the ring from without. 3. A ring (*D*) to protect the forefinger.

The process is quite a recent one, and has not as yet been attended with any very great success. Bouchut reports seven cases, five of which terminated fatally, and the other two underwent tracheotomy. At a meeting of the French Academy of Medicine, a committee was appointed to examine M. Bouchut's communication on the subject; of this committee M. Trousseau was appointed

Fig. 3.

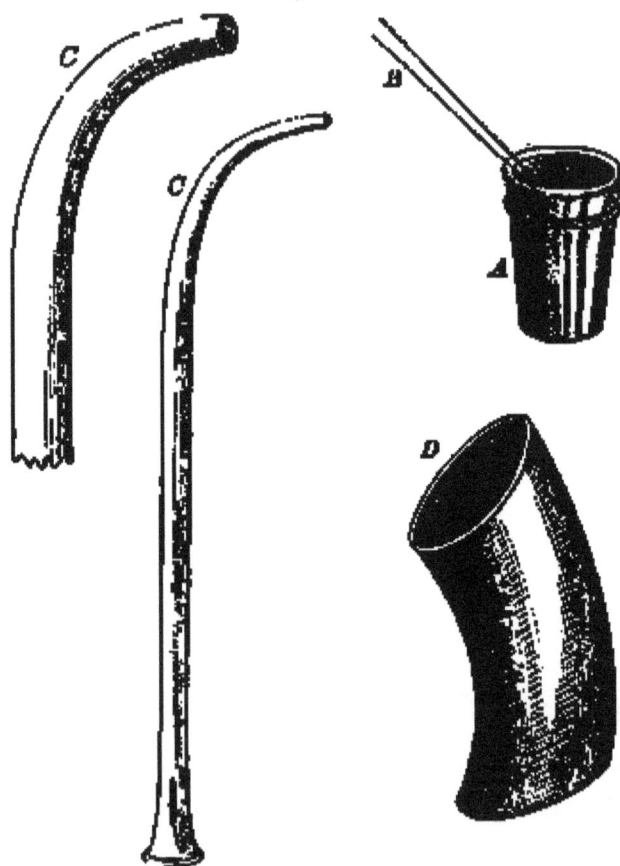

chairman. The report, which is of some length, concludes with the following resolutions:—

"1. Tubing the larynx, in certain forms of acute laryngitis, may, by delaying asphyxia, become a remedial agent.

"2. In certain chronic affections of the same organ,

tubing may permit tracheotomy to be postponed, and
may occasionally give time to treat and cure the disease.

"3. In the treatment of croup, tubing retards asphyxia,
and affords a more easy mode of introduction into the air-
passages of remedies calculated to modify diphtheritic
inflammation.

"4. It cannot, however, supply the place of tracheotomy, which to this day remains the only expedient in
croup, when the resources of medicine seem to have been
exhausted."

RÉSUMÉ.

In the preceding pages, we first gave Bretonneau's
description of diphtheria. We then remarked that it
was only by a comparison of the various epidemics of
"sore throat" which had prevailed at intervals in various
parts of the world, that we could ascertain how far his
description was to be taken as a model of the disease.
Accordingly we took up the history of the epidemics
from remote ages to the present day.

Having given an account of those which had prevailed
in various parts of Europe, and having compared the
descriptions of various writers upon these epidemics,
with that of Bretonneau, we showed that he was incorrect
in denying the presence of all constitutional disturbance,
as also in insisting upon the absence of all relation between diphtheria and gangrene of the fauces—both of
these conditions having been frequently observed, particularly during the epidemics of late years.

We next observed that Bretonneau's idea of croup, which he associates with diphtheria, does not conform to our ideas of that disease, founded, as they are, upon the description given by Dr. Home. The distinctions between diphtheria and croup were dwelt upon, as also the non-identity of diphtheria and scarlatina.

In order, we took up the history of the disease in England. A comparison of the descriptions of the disease by various writers, as it appeared in the several counties, gave no marked uniformity, and but little correspondence with Bretonneau's model.

Diphtheria in America was then considered, and we gave at some length a description of an epidemic of "sore throat," by Dr. Bard, also an account of the epidemics in California and other parts of the Union.

We next remarked that all these epidemics of "sore throat" were connected by a bond of union, to be found in the pathological anatomy of the disease, which consists in the peculiar exudation. That although Bretonneau fully recognized this fact, his description was deficient, hence we subjoined that of MM. Barthez and Rilliet, as being more comprehensive. We also considered the disease as existing under two forms, the mild and severe.

Certain points as respects the nature of the disease were taken up in order. First, the characteristics of the false membrane, its physical appearances, its seat, the experiments of Bretonneau in order to ascertain the specific nature of the diphtheritic membrane, its microscopic appearances, and its dependence upon certain parasites were discussed.

Next, in answer to the question, Is diphtheria infectious? Having given the arguments of various authors, we replied, that although we were ignorant of the exact laws which governed these epidemics, we are able to detect certain hygienic or individual circumstances which undoubtedly had their effect, either as direct or as predisposing causes.

The presence of albumen in the urine and its signification were commented upon. We remarked that further observation*was necessary before we could ascribe to it any settled prognostic value. We spoke of the singular after-effects of the disease, as shown especially upon the nervous system. We gave the observations of MM. Trousseau, Faure, and others upon this point.

In our account of the *treatment* of diphtheria, we said that it was only within the last few years that anything like unanimity had prevailed. That it was now universally regarded as an asthenic disease, and consequently would bear no depletory measures, but, on the contrary, required tonics, stimulants, and a nourishing diet, even in the early stages. Blisters, leeches, and local bleeding of any sort should be prohibited.

The tonics best suited we enumerated. Of the auxiliary measures, we first spoke of the local applications to the fauces, their utility and propriety, the various agents which had been employed and the mode of use. The ablation of the tonsils recommended by Bouchut, we con-

ceived to be inadmissible, excepting under rare circumstances.

Tracheotomy we discussed at considerable length.
Remarking that the two diseases, inflammatory croup
and diphtheria, were on an equal footing as regards the
applicability of the operation, we answered the various
objections which had been brought against it; the small
amount of success; the difficulties of performing it; the
tendency to the production of bronchitis, &c.

We considered that the proper time for performing
the operation was an intermediate period. We gave some
necessary rules as to the size of the canula, the state of
the surrounding atmosphere, the importance of having
some competent person at hand in the case of emergency,
the propriety of keeping up the medical treatment, and
the time for removing the canula.

Having given a summary of the treatment recommended by some of the leading men in Europe, we
concluded by a brief consideration of the operation for
"tubing the larynx."

www.ingramcontent.com/pod-product-compliance
Lightning Source LLC
Chambersburg PA
CBHW021812190326
41518CB00007B/556